Weight-Watchers Freestyle Cookbook

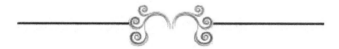

This Diet Book Includes Quick and Easy Healthy Recipes And a 3-Week Weight Loss Plan. It Also Explains Weight-Watchers Smart Points System and How to Use Instant Pot Slow Cook

Table of Contents

—⁓⁕⁓—

Introduction

Have you found yourself in a difficult situation, wondering what your next steps should be? Have you tried many different ways to lose weight and get healthy, only to find yourself falling off track again and again? You are not alone, as many people find themselves in the exact same situation, time, and time again. This can feel disheartening, and it can leave you feeling like a failure, but I assure you that there are far more people in this situation today than you think.

Thank you for choosing this book. Throughout these pages, we will look at the Weight Watchers diet in detail, including the lifestyle changes that should accompany this type of diet change in order to set you up for the most success possible.

Whether you have experience with Weight Watchers, or you are completely new to the concept of it, we will begin from square one so that you are given a foundation from which to build the life and body of your dreams.

This diet has been around for some time now, and it has evolved over the years to be able to fit with the lives of the modern father, mother, professional, and so on. Whoever you are this diet will fit with your life and will be able to keep you on track to becoming the best version of yourself that you could possibly imagine!

Chapter 1: What Is Weight Watchers?

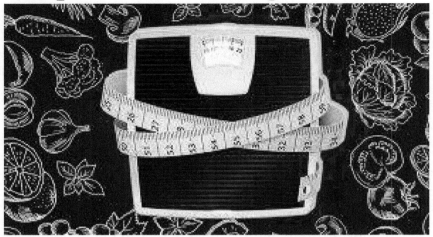

Welcome to chapter one, where we will discuss the origins of Weight Watchers and what it was designed for. To begin, I will talk about what Weight Watchers is and a background of its history.

What Is Weight Watchers?

Weight Watchers is both a company and a diet program, which has been around for some time now. When it was first introduced, it came as a new way of dieting that simplified food consumption into categories of foods that were allowed to be eaten in an unlimited amount, foods that were limited, and foods that were completely restricted.

Now, since it has evolved over the years, it aims to be known as a different way to view food consumption, and which wanted to show people that a diet plan should be more than just a restrictive way of eating, but that instead, it should be a new lifestyle altogether. Weight Watchers wanted to show people that they can still enjoy life while trying to lose weight and get healthy.

The History of Weight Watchers

Weight Watchers began in the 1960s in New York City, USA, when the founder wanted to brainstorm new ideas and methods for losing weight. It was this brainstorming that first led to the inception of Weight Watchers. This happened in the early sixties, and by 1968 the founder- named Jean Nidetch, had created a company that was generating a large amount of income and that had developed into an incorporated brand. When it began, the rules of the weight loss program were quite strict when it came to telling participants what they could and could not eat. Some examples of this extreme restriction included completely cutting out avocadoes, peanut butter, bananas, watermelon, cherries, yogurt and bacon, among others, and ensuring that the participants ate fish no less than five times per week. The company went public in 1968 and Nidetch's earnings reached a new high.

As the years went on, the diet plan evolved with time, and it became less restrictive than in its beginnings. This is likely because it changed hands and was sold to the Heinz brand, the same Heinz as the ketchup manufacturers in 1978. At that point, it was worth 71 million dollars. The one thing that most people know about weight watchers is that it uses a points system. We will look into the most modern version of this point system in more detail soon, but when it began, the points system involved all foods being assigned a points value based on their calorie content. This allowed participants to choose their foods based on their assigned point value, which ensured that they were sticking within their predetermined daily calorie intake values. This initial point system came about in 1997, about thirty years after the beginning of Weight Watchers.

Weight Watchers was sold again in 1999, to an investment company based in Europe.

In the year 2000, Weight Watchers once again changed, removing the food restrictions and instead focusing on calorie intake based on the points awarded to specific foods. This new system included more individualized programming and adjustments according to exercise levels. This new evolution of the program was a better fit for the lifestyles of individuals and ventured away from a one size fits all approach. This new program had a better understanding of weight loss and calorie intake, as well as the mental toll that restricting certain foods altogether took on people, leading them to fall off track or abandon the diet plan altogether. By allowing certain foods to be eaten that were previously restricted, this helped people who experienced severe cravings to continue to follow the plan while giving into their cravings every now and then in order to help them remain in a good headspace.

In the year 2004, the program evolved again, allowing participants to choose one of two program options. The first was a program that involved foods deemed compliant, and others deemed non-compliant, which did not include point values anymore. The second was a system that still included points, but that did not restrict foods, only requested that people stick within their specific points values. This allowed people to eat anything they wanted, but they had to remain within specific calorie goals each day.

In 2008, a new program was developed that combined both of the previous plan options into one new plan called the *Momentum Plan,* which stuck to the points system but that did not restrict foods. Instead, it guided participants toward specific foods that were better choices than others.

Just two short years later in 2010, the entire program saw an overhaul, which included a new way of looking at foods for more than just the number of calories they contained. IN the previous program, people could eat anything they wanted as long as it fits within their calorie goals, but this meant that they were not always making the healthiest choices for their overall health. This new program in 2010 brought insight into the nutritional value that certain foods offered, including their content of protein, fat and fiber content.

Later on, in 2015, more emphasis was placed on exercise, and this allowed people to incorporate points called *FitPoints* which accounted for people's calorie expenditure during exercise and which then affected their calorie intake for the day.

In 2017, the newest program was announced, which is still used to this day. This plan is called WW Freestyle. This is the plan that we will look at in more detail throughout this book.

The most recent change in the company- in 2018 brought a new name, where Weight Watchers became "WW International Inc." With this change in title came a change in philosophy and values, as WW began to focus more on wellness than on weight loss. This is likely due to the change in culture, as society at this time is more focused on overall life satisfaction than on reaching a goal weight or a small pant size. With the changing of the world, Weight Watchers has evolved in order to continue to serve both women and men in the most effective ways possible. As much more emphasis is placed on leading a healthy, active and fulfilling life now more than ever, Weight Watchers has grown to take this into account, helping people to become the healthiest version of themselves so that they feel happier and more confident overall.

Weight Watchers holds meetings in various locations around the world in order to give people an opportunity to come together and hear experts speak, get support from others who are following the program, and gain motivation to continue their healthy lifestyle by seeing Weight Watchers Lifetime Members who have been with the brand for many, many years.

What Is the Philosophy Behind Weight Watchers?

The philosophy of Weight Watchers is, at its core, to help people maintain weight management in a healthy and lasting way. Weight Watchers believes that dieting is only one part of the weight management equation and that it must also include mental wellbeing and emotional wellbeing. Weight Watchers believes that weight management comes from a healthy lifestyle and it aims to help participants achieve this in the simplest and most effective way possible. Instead of telling people what they can and cannot do, Weight Watchers gives participants information and guidance regarding exercise, nutrition and dieting. Weight Watchers encourages people to find fun and enjoyable ways to achieve a healthy lifestyle, whatever that looks like to them specifically.

How WW Can Benefit You

There are a variety of ways in which Weight Watchers will benefit you. The most recent form of Weight Watchers will provide you with the following benefits,

- It is flexible, so it can easily fit into your current lifestyle, which will increase your chances of sticking to the program and seeing lasting results.
- Weight Watchers incorporates exercise and adjusts your calorie allowance based on this
- Weight Watchers will help you to see slow and steady weight loss, so that the weight stays off
- Weight Watchers offers you the best methods for lasting results
- Weight Watchers is well-established, so it offers a wealth of resources and support for its participants
- Weight Watchers does not limit any foods completely, which increases the chances of sticking to the diet
- Weight Watchers teaches excellent habits and will help you to grow lifelong habits that will continue to benefit you for years to come.
- There are countless testimonials from past participants and a wealth of people to give advice who have been through the program.

What Is WW Good For?

Weight Watchers is a great way for people who have been trying various weight loss programs and diet programs but who have had difficulty sticking to a program, or who have had trouble keeping the weight off after initially seeing results. Weight Watchers aims to help you develop a completely new lifestyle so that you are able to view weight loss as a way of life rather than a crash-course. In order to lose

7

weight and keep weight off, it is necessary to lead a healthy and active lifestyle, and Weight Watchers will help guide you as you begin to make changes toward this type of lifestyle.

WW is great for anybody who thinks that they are too busy to follow a diet plan, too busy to meal prep or too busy to change any aspect of their life. Since it uses a point system, it could not be easier to begin changing your diet and your lifestyle as a whole.

What Are Smart Points?

The data behind diet and weight loss programs can be overwhelming and quite complicated for those who do not have a background in nutritional science- which is almost all of us! By using a points system, WW breaks down this complex information into small, easy to understand numerical values, which means that anybody can take control of their diet and their weight loss without having to study for years to understand it all!

Every food has a Smart Points value. This value has been determined by experts in the field of dieting and nutrition. In order to properly understand the Smart Points values that the foods you eat have been assigned, you must understand at least a basic level of food and nutrition science. In this section, we will look at Smart Points while learning about what some of the components in our food are called, and what they mean.

Benefits of Smart Points- Based Eating

One of the great things about this diet is that it is not one that is founded on restricting a person's intake heavily and only allowing a small number of foods. Diets like this that work by heavily restricting food intake are extremely hard to transition to and fit into a person's lifestyle, and they are hard to maintain for a long period of time.

The Weight Watchers diet is about including as many natural, plant-based foods as you wish, while also not excluding things like lean meats or fish and even some treats now and then. This makes it much easier to stick with this type of diet and reduces the chances of falling off after a short period of time due to cravings or intense hunger. It does not restrict calories or reduce your intake greatly, which makes it easier to handle for many. It feels natural to eat in this way, which makes it effective.

The Basics of Weight Loss

First though, we will discuss weight loss as a general concept. The most basic concept of weight loss is that you must put your body in a calorie deficit for your body to lose weight in the form of fat. What this means is that you must eat fewer calories than you burn, which will result in a loss of weight. The equation for this concept is below;

The number of calories that you ingest **– (minus)** The number of calories you use to survive (for example, walking, eating, breathing) **– (minus)** The extra calories burned from exercise = **(equals) = + (positive) or – (negative)**

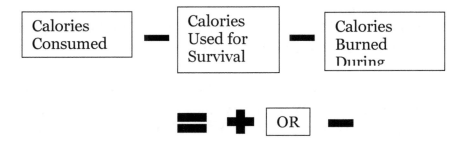

The number that results from this equation will be either positive or negative. This will mean one of three things.

1. If the number is positive, this means that you ingested more calories than you burned.
2. If the number is negative, this means that you burned more calories than you ingested.
3. If the number is zero, this means that calories ingested, and calories burned are equal to one another.

If the number is zero, this indicates "breaking even" in terms of your energy. If the number is positive, you can envision it like having more energy than you were able to use. When this occurs, the extra energy is stored as fat in the body. If the number is negative, you used more energy than you had, and this translates to weight loss, as once the energy is all used up, the fat stores will begin to be used for additional energy.

The key to weight loss is attaining a negative number of calories each day. This will mean that you are burning slightly more calories than you ingest each day, meaning that over time you will lose a small amount of weight each day, and this will add up to create a steady weight loss over time.

This steady weight loss over time is the goal of the Weight Watchers program. Instead of having to calculate all of your calories each day and determine how many calories you burned in order to determine if you are at a caloric deficit, the Weight Watchers Smart Points have done this for you.

What Are Macronutrients?

To begin, we are going to look at how a person would come to understand their own personal daily intake of macronutrients. *Macronutrients* are those nutrients within food that are comprised of other, smaller nutrients. These macronutrients are those components of food that you have no doubt heard of before, such as the following,

- Carbohydrates
- Protein
- Fat.

These macronutrients are the things that you will often hear about when a scientist would be talking about a food's health content, or about its level of "healthiness." These three macronutrients come together to form the calorie content of a food item.

The Weight Watchers Smart Points system follows the following general structure when determining the number of points a food item contains. The calories of a food will determine the starting value. Once the starting value has been established, there will be adjustments made depending on the macronutrient content. The protein content will lower the smart point value. Sugar and Saturated Fats will increase the Smart Points value. The reason for this is that there have been studies done that have shown that eating more protein as well as less Sugar and Saturated Fats will lead to better chances of weight loss as well as a healthier overall life and body.

It is important to get an idea of what your own personal number of calories- as well as fat and protein intake should be so that you can determine if you are eating enough, too much or just the right amount. This is helpful when it comes to weight loss. When following the WW program, this is done for you based on a series of questions about your life and your body. If you know what your regular daily intake should be, this tells you the number of calories that you would need to eat in order to maintain your weight exactly where it is currently. Then, in order to lose weight, Weight Watchers reduces this number of calories slightly, so that you will be put into a calorie deficit each day, resulting in weight loss over time. Your caloric intake does not need to be severely restricted to the point where you are feeling hungry all of the time, in order to do this, it is only necessary to put yourself into a small deficit and this will lead you to lose weight over time.

This calorie calculation is based on age, sex, height, weight, and activity level, as all of these factors influence your body's use of calories per day and the amount of each macronutrient in particular that you should be ingesting.

To begin, Weight Watchers will calculate your BMR or Basal Metabolic Rate. This is an indicator of the number of calories your body needs in order to simply live. This includes breathing, talking, moving, and so on, without any exercise. The bigger the person's body, the more calories they will need to maintain life. The reason that this calculation takes age into consideration is that as we get older, our amount of muscle generally decreases. Thus, we must take this into account as this reduces the number of calories needed to run our body's functions. Further, there is a different calculation for men than for women, as male bodies and female bodies use energy differently.

The next factor that will go into the Weight Watchers method of calculating your daily intake is to determine your TDEE or your Total Daily Energy Expenditure. This number will tell you how much energy your body uses on a daily basis, including your exercise. While BMR tells you how much energy you use if you were to just live for a day without spending any extra energy, TDEE will give you a more realistic number as it will include your level of activity.

Now that we know the number of calories your body uses in one average day, you can adjust this amount in order to put yourself in a caloric deficit, which will lead to weight loss. If you want to maintain your weight, you will eat exactly as many calories as you need in order to sustain your life and activity level (TDEE). If, however, you want to lose weight, this is what you will do. In order to begin losing weight, the recommended caloric reduction is between 10 and 20%. It is not advised to reduce your caloric intake by any more than 30%, as this can leave you without enough energy to sustain your regular activity and daily life.

Once this calculation has been determined, Weight Watchers will give you a point value, which represents your daily allowance of Smart Points. Weight Watchers will also allow you some extra smart points each week in order to account for those special occasions or specific days when you need a few extra points to work with. This is called your own personalized Smart Points daily or weekly Budget.

Further, if there are Smart Points at the end of the day that you have not used, meaning that you have some calories that you have left over that have not been ingested, you can take these into the rest of the week. These calories or Smart Points that are left over are called *Rollovers*. You can take up to 4 Smart Points per day into your weekly Rollover allowance. These can be used later on in the week if you have a meal that is higher in calories than you would usually choose, or if you have a special occasion on the weekend that you need a few extra points for. These extra Smart Points, along with your extra weekly Smart Point allowance can be used all at once for an extra special meal, they can be used a little at a time or you can split them up however else you wish to. This allows for flexibility and it allows you to continue living, instead of having to halt your life altogether in order to change your life and your body!

WW Smartphone Applications

My WW
There is a Weight Watchers specific application for your smartphone that will help you to keep track of your smart points throughout the day and determine the number of Smart Points for specific foods. This application also tracks your rollover allowance and can tell you how many Smart Points you have left for the week and for the end of the day. This application is simply called *My WW*. You can find this application in the app store on your phone, and you can begin tracking and noting your point values right away.

In this application, you can also track your activity levels, your weekly allowance, you can engage and interact with other participants who are also using the application, and you can even scan food packaging that you purchase in the grocery store to determine the Smart Points value of the foods you are shopping for.

Ultimate Value Diary
This is another application for smartphones that helps you to track and calculate your daily intake and your weekly remaining points value. It also keeps track of your exercise and accounts for this in your calorie allowance.

Nutrition Menu
This application is a little different than the two above, as it aims to help you determine the calorie content and point values for restaurants and fast food outlets. This is helpful for those who travel often, as it can help you to navigate the menu, which can prove to be quite difficult if it presents you with foods that you are not used to eating on your new Weight Watchers Smart Points plan.

Chapter 2: Weight Watchers Freestyle

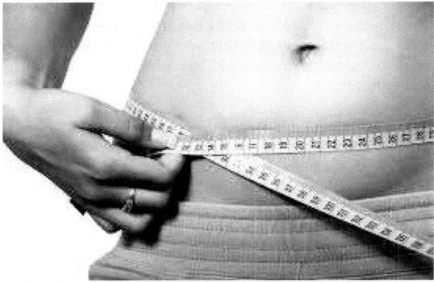

In this chapter, we will delve into WW Freestyle, which is the newest version of the Weight Watchers plan to date. This plan is more tailored and allows for more flexibility, making it a great choice for many people because of its ease of incorporation into a variety of lifestyles. We will begin looking at what exactly WW Freestyle is, and then we will look at more specific food allowances on this program.

What Is WW Freestyle?

Weight Watchers, or WW Freestyle, is the newest version of the Weight Watchers brand of diet plans. This new Freestyle plan has been tailored and changed over time in order to eventually come up with this plan- the most flexible and effective to date. On WW Freestyle, there are no foods that are off-limits, no foods that you must completely stay away from. Many other diet plans focus on restriction, but this WW program does not, as it understands that restriction is one of the fastest ways to have people fall off of the wagon when it comes to dieting.

Further, there are some foods which are called *Zero Point Foods*. These foods have been determined to have a zero-point value, because of their ratio of protein versus calories. These foods are dense in nutrients and low in calories, which makes them great options for a healthy body and lifestyle. Any time you eat mostly plant-sourced foods or foods that are closer to their natural state, they will contain high amounts of fiber and a large water content, especially in the case of vegetables. This means that people who eat a diet rich in these foods will feel more full earlier than those who do not and will remain full for longer. This is because of the high fiber and the high content of water, which fills a person's stomach much quicker than other foods would. These Zero Points Foods can be eaten in unlimited amounts without being logged or tracked in any way, as they do not take away from your daily or weekly point value allowance. Later on, in this chapter, we will look at some of these foods that have a zero-point value.

How Do Smart Points Come Into Play in the Freestyle Program?

Each individual that takes part in WW Freestyle will be given somewhere between 30 and 45 Smart Points per day. Below is a list of some common foods and their WW Smart Points values. This will help you when determining which foods you want to include in your diet each day and what the foods that you normally eat look like in terms of their Smart Points Values.

17

- 1 Ounce of Tortilla chips: 4 Smart Points
- Fat-Free Salsa: 0 Smart Points
- 1 Tbsp Olive oil: 4 Smart Points
- Mayonnaise: (1 Tbsp) 3 Smart Points
- Half & half Cream: (2 tbsp) 2 Smart Points
- 1 tsp white Sugar: 1 Point
- Guacamole: (2 Tbsp) 1 Smart Point
- Salad: (mixed greens) 0 Smart Points
- Rice, brown: (cooked, 1 cup) 6 Smart Points
- Shrimp: (cooked, 3 oz.) 1 Smart Point
- 1 cup Cooked Oatmeal: 5 Points
- Mustard: 0 Points
- Splenda: (1-3 packets) 0 WW points
- Lettuce: (Romaine, iceberg) 0 SmartPoints
- Mushrooms: 0 SmartPoints
- 1 C One Percent Milk: 4 Points
- Bread, 1 slice: 2 Points
- B1 serving light beer: 5 Smart Points
- Butter: (1 tbsp) 5 Smart Points
- Celery: 0 Smart Points
- Strawberries: 0 Smart Points
- Black beans, 1/2 C: 3 Points
- Banana: 0 Smart Points
- 4.5 ounce beef hamburger, no bun: 8 Smart Points
- Hamburger bun: 5 Smart Points
- Spinach: 0 Smart Points
- Cherries: 0 Smart Points

- 1/2C mashed Potatoes:4 Points
- 1C Rice, white: 6 Smart Points
- 1C unsweetened almond milk: 1 Point
- 1 Tbsp honey: 4 Smart Points
- ¼ Avocado: 2 Smart Points
- 3oz canned tuna: 1 Point
- 3 ounces cooked ground beef (90%): 4 Points
- 3 ounce vegetarian burger: 3 Smart Points
- ½ cup Sweet Potatoes: 3 Smart Points
- 2 Tbsp peanut butter: 6 Smart Points
- English muffin: 4 Smart Points
- Onions: 0 Smart Points
- 1 med. Size flour tortilla: 3 Smart Points
- Scrambled eggs with butter & milk: 6 Smart Points
- Corn on the cob: 4 Smart Points
- Carrots: 0 Smart Point
- Diet Coke, 12 oz. (0 SP)
- 12 oz. Soda Pop: 7 Smart Points
- Asparagus: 0 Smart Points
- Caesar salad: (3 cups) 10 Smart Points
- Wine, Red: (5 oz) 4 Smart Points
- Plain greek yogurt: 0 Smart Points
- Blueberries: 0 Smart Points
- Orange Juice: 6 Smart Points
- 3 ounce tuna steak: 1 Smart Point
- 1 Hard-boiled egg: 2 Smart Points
- 2 ounces deli turkey: 1 Smart Point

19

- Tomatoes: (Regular, grape, cherry) 0 Smart Points
- Peach: 0 Smart Points
- Milk, whole: (1 cup) 7 Smart Points
- 1 Cup Plain yogurt: 3 Smart Points
- Plain baked potato: 5 Smart Points
- 1 Cup Pasta: 5 Smart Points
- 1 Cup Skim milk: 3 Smart Points
- 2 ounces deli ham: 2 Smart Points
- Egg, fried: 3 Smart Points
- Balsamic vinaigrette dressing: 1 Smart Point
- Pear: 0 Smart Points
- Black coffee: 0 Smart Points
- Pineapple: 0 Smart Points
- Tilapia fish: 1 Smart Point
- Raspberries: 0 Smart Points
- Turkey burger & bun: 9 Smart Points
- Broccoli: 0 Smart Points
- 20 French fries: 13 Smart Points
- 1 ounce feta cheese: 3 Smart Points
- Green beans: 0 SmartPoints
- Turkey bacon: (cooked, 3 slices) 3 Smart Points
- ¼ C Cheddar cheese: 4 Smart Points
- Cantaloupe: 0 Smart Points
- Apple: 0 Smart Points
- Red peppers: 0 Smart Points
- 3 ounce chicken breast: 2 Smart Points
- Bagel: 5 Smart Points
- Pizza: (slice) That depends... 7-12 Smart Points

- Egg white: 0 Smart Points
- Watermelon: 0 Smart Points
- Hummus: 2 Smart Points
- Cookie: 3 Smart Points
- Cheeseburger with bun: 12 Smart Points

- ¼ Cup Almonds: Smart Points
- 3 ounce pork chop: 3 Smart Points
- Wine, white: (5 ounces) 4 Smart Points
- Bacon: (cooked, 3 slices) 5 Smart Points
- Salmon: (wild-caught) 0 points

As you can see from the comprehensive list above, the foods that are less nutritious will come with higher Smart Point values, and the foods that are more nutritionally dense (in terms of their vitamins, minerals, and overall nutrients) will come with much lower Smart Points values. You may have noticed that some of the foods on the list above have a Zero Smart Points value. You may be wondering how this could be possible? In the next section, we will look at foods that have a Zero Smart Points value and what this means for your WW Freestyle diet.

Foods That Have Zero Smart Points

Vegetables contain low numbers of calories and carbohydrates but have many beneficial vitamins and minerals. The body does not digest fiber, so it is good to eat vegetables that contain fiber as they help you to feel full without actually filling your body with digestible carbohydrates. When looking at which vegetables to eat, take the total amount of carbohydrates and subtract from it the amount of fiber to find out how many carbs your body will actually absorb from it.

Vegetables have a very low-calorie content for their size, which means that they will fill your stomach without giving you a large calorie count. Because of this, when you become full by eating a salad, for example, you will not be able to eat any more food, but you will not have ingested a large number of calories. This can lead to a calorie deficit and subsequent weight loss if this type of eating is continued.

Plant-Based Zero Point Foods

The foods contained in this list can be said to be a comprehensive list of what a plant-based diet or a plant-based The Weight Watcher Freestyle program encourages a plant-based style of eating, which is nutrient-dense and will provide you with the fuel and energy your body needs to be a healthy and well-functioning machine. If you are unsure of what a plant-based diet is, we will look at that here in this section before I share with you the zero-point foods included in the WW Freestyle program.

A plant-based diet is a style of eating that is focused on only plant-forward sources of food. This is not only restricted to vegetables and fruits, but any other plant sources of food as well. This style of eating does not mean the same thing as being vegetarian or vegan, and it does not say anything about what you can eat in terms of meat and dairy. However, there are many similarities to a vegetarian style of eating or a Mediterranean style of eating. A Mediterranean style of eating comes from the foods that would commonly be eaten by people who reside around the Mediterranean. Thus it includes foods that would be grown and found in these regions. Many of these foods are plant-based, but it also includes fish, poultry and dairy in small quantities. This is one example of a style of eating that is mostly plant-based but that is not vegetarian or vegan.

A vegetarian diet, however, is also another example of a diet that can be mostly plant-based, but without including meats. However, a vegetarian diet is not always plant-based if the individual eats a high amount of processed foods.

The plant-based style of eating can be flexible and tailored to the specific individual, which is one of its benefits. This diet is focused on keeping foods as natural as possible and avoiding heavily processed foods.

One of the added benefits of plant-based eating, such as the style of eating that is encouraged by the WW Freestyle program, is that it is not only beneficial for a person's body and their health, but it is also beneficial for the environment. By reducing the amount of processed foods that you eat, you are reducing your carbon footprint as the factories that produce these foods use a lot of energy and resources which leads to pollution of the environment. Since one of the main factors of a plant-based diet is that it involves whole and natural foods, the foods you will be eating are ingested as close to the state in which they are found in nature as possible, which is better for the environment and will help you do your part for the environment while also improving your health!

The following list is a comprehensive list of foods that are attributed the number Zero Points as a Value in the WW Freestyle diet plan, and which are what make up a healthy and well-rounded plant-based diet.

Beans & Legumes

Frozen, fresh, or even canned legumes and beans that are free from sugars and/or oils. These include:

- Black beans
- fat-free refried beans
- split peas
- navy beans
- kidney beans
- great northern beans
- pinto beans
- chickpeas,
- fava beans
- black-eyed peas
- lima beans
- soybeans
- lentils
- edamame
- kidney beans
- Adzuki beans

Chicken & Turkey Breast

These include:

- skinless chicken breast
- skinless turkey breast
- ground turkey
- ground chicken

Eggs

These include:

- Egg yolks
- whole eggs
- Egg whites
- egg substitutes

Fish & Shellfish

These include all kinds of frozen, fresh, smoked and canned (in water or sauce) fish or shellfish including:

- Langoustine
- Lobster
- Oysters
- Crab
- Salmon
- Clams
- Crayfish
- Tuna
- Barnacles
- Mussels
- Shark
- Snails
- Octopus
- Land snails
- Squid
- Sea bream
- Shrimps
- Krill
- Cod
- Scallops
- Prawn
- Haddock
- Cuttlefish
- Trout

Fruits

Frozen and fresh fruit including canned fruit in water or sugar-free syrup, canned fruit in its own natural juice, and unsweetened applesauce *without any added sugar* (however, this excludes dried fruits and fruit juices). Some examples include:

- Tropical fruits including bananas and mangoes
- Citrus fruits such as oranges, grapefruits, mandarins and limes
- Melons including watermelons, rock melons, and honeydew melons
- Berries such as passionfruit, strawberries, kiwi fruit, raspberries, blueberries
- Apples and pears
- Stone fruit such as plums, peaches, apricots
- Other fruits such as tomatoes and avocados

Plain Nonfat Yogurt & Plain Soy Yogurt

- Plain greek yogurt, plain yogurt, soy yogurt, plain quark

Tofu & Tempeh

- Firm tofu
- Soft or silken tofu
- Smoked tofu
- Tempeh cooked in a variety of ways

Starchy Vegetables

- Frozen, fresh or canned starchy vegetables including,
- succotash
- parsnips
- split peas

- corn
- green peas

Non-Starchy Vegetables

These can be in the form of fresh, canned or even frozen vegetables with no added salt or flavorings.

- Swiss chard
- Asparagus
- Turnips
- Cauliflower
- Brussels sprouts
- Beets
- Jicama
- Daikon
- Squash varieties including spaghetti squash, crookneck, cushaw, zucchini squash, and summer squash
- Artichoke
- Sprouts
- Artichoke hearts
- Cabbages such as Chinese cabbage, green cabbage, bok choy
- Onions
- Mushrooms
- Leeks
- Tomato
- Cucumber
- Water chestnuts
- Yard-long beans
- Carrots
- Bamboo shoots
- Salad greens such as spinach, chicory greens, radicchio, lettuce, endives, escarole, romaine, arugula, watercress
- Eggplant
- Greens such as collard,

- turnip, kale, and mustard
- Okra
- Broccoli
- Amaranth or Chinese spinach
- Peppers such as jalapeno peppers and bell peppers
- Celery
- Beans (green beans, wax beans, Italian beans)
- Radishes
- Hearts of palm
- Peapods
- Baby corn
- Chayote
- Rutabaga
- Kohlrabi
- Sugar snap peas
- Bean sprouts
- Coleslaw (packaged and with no dressing)

Zero Point Value Condiments and Seasonings

- Soy sauce
- Hot sauce
- Fresh and dried herbs and spices
- Lemon, lime or orange zest
- Wine vinegars
- Mustard
- Lemon or lime juice
- Fat-free salsa
- Unsweetened pickles

Exceptions to the Zero Points Value Rules

There are some exceptions to these zero-point value foods. This is due to the fact that some of the foods on this list are high in calories and are lower in fiber than the others that are included in the zero points list.

- Potatoes
- Yams and Sweet Potatoes
- Olives
- Avocados
- Vegetable Flours such as squash flour, pumpkin flour, potato flour, and carrot flour

When it comes to the foods that you choose to eat, you will want to ensure that you are choosing as many foods as you can that are included in the Zero Points Value list. This will help you to not only feel full and increase your chances of weight loss, but it will help to improve the health of your body from the inside so that you can begin to decrease your risk of disease and improve the overall functioning of your body.

Chapter 3: WW Freestyle 3 Week Plan

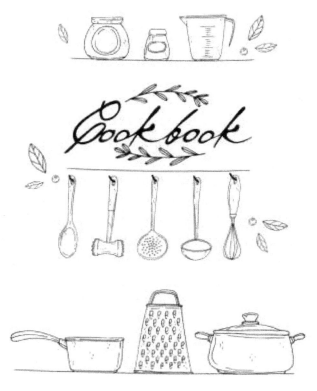

In this chapter, we are going to look at how you can begin your first three weeks on the WW diet plan. As the first few weeks will likely be the most challenging for you, it will be beneficial to have a plan to follow so that you don't have to try to figure out each day's meal plan while you are hungry and still adjusting to the new lifestyle that you have undertaken. To begin, I will lay out a shopping guide for you, and then you can see how this would come together in a meal plan and, in the next chapter, in a recipe booklet.

WW Freestyle Shopping Guide

- Ground chicken breast
- Salad greens such as spinach, chicory greens, radicchio, lettuce, endives, escarole, romaine, arugula, watercress or any others that you enjoy
- Cabbages such as Chinese cabbage, green cabbage or Bok Choy
- Firm Tofu
- Prawns or Shrimp
- Cucumbers
- Chickpeas
- Clams
- Watermelon or Honeydew melon
- Fava beans
- Skinless chicken breast
- Peas in their pods
- Water Chestnuts
- Artichoke Hearts
- Beets
- Boneless, Skinless Turkey Breast
- Tomato
- Unsweetened Pickles
- Scallops
- Fresh and dried herbs and spices
- Swiss chard
- Squid
- Egg whites
- Baby corn
- black-eyed peas
- Mushrooms
- Radishes
- Lemons
- Apples and Pears
- Asparagus
- Avocado
- Crayfish

31

- Citrus fruits such as oranges, grapefruits, and mandarin oranges
- Parsnips
- Artichokes
- Stone fruit such as plums, peaches, apricots
- Oysters
- Soybeans
- Tempeh cooked in a variety of ways
- Tuna
- Other fruits such as tomatoes and avocados
- Plain non-fat Greek yogurt
- Trout Fish
- Lobster
- Coleslaw (packaged and with no dressing)
- Sprouts
- Salmon
- Sugar snap peas
- Amaranth or Chinese spinach
- Great Northern Beans
- Mustard
- Cod Fish
- Lentils
- Cuttlefish
- Spaghetti squash or Summer Squash
- corn
- Fat-Free Refried Beans
- Berries such as passionfruit, strawberries, kiwi fruit, raspberries, blueberries
- Daikon
- pinto beans
- Wine vinegars
- Greens such as collard, turnip, kale and mustard greens
- Kohlrabi

32

- Lima Beans
- Limes
- Turnips
- Whole, Omega-3 Fortified Eggs
- Fat-Free Salsa
- Split Peas
- Carrots
- Celery
- Eggplant
- Ground Turkey Breast
- Soy sauce
- Bean sprouts
- Peppers such as jalapeno peppers
- and bell peppers
- Bamboo shoots
- Leeks
- Lamb
- Pork Chops
- Frozen, fresh or canned starchy vegetables
- Onions
- Linguine
- Other types of beans (kidney beans, green beans, wax beans, Italian beans,
- Yard-long beans
- Black beans)
- Brussels Sprouts
- Haddock Fish
- Cauliflower
- Langoustine
- Okra
- Rutabaga
- Tropical fruits including bananas and mangoes
- Mussels
- Broccoli
- Edamame

Shopping Guide Tips and Tricks

In this section, we will look at how to approach the grocery store. When you are entering the grocery store, it is important that you do a few different things to prepare yourself, especially when beginning a new diet as it will be challenging for you to enter the grocery store when you are having cravings and temptations while you adjust to your new diet plan. The following tips will guide you through your first number of grocery shopping experiences while you navigate this new diet.

- **Don't Go to the Grocery Store When You Are Hungry**

One of the biggest things that are important to mention to everyone when beginning any sort of new diet is to never shop when you are hungry. Shopping when you are hungry will make you reach for anything and everything that you see on the shelves. By entering the grocery store when you are full or when you have just eaten, you will be able to stick to your list and avoid falling prey to temptations, which will keep you on track in terms of your diet and eating the foods that you have planned rather than those impulse items that you want to reach for in times of hunger. This is the easiest way to slip back into your old ways.

- **Avoid Temptations While You Shop**

If you are going to be eating a plant-focused diet, you will be spending the majority of your time while in the grocery store around the outer perimeter of the store. This is where the whole foods and plant-based foods are located. By doing this, and entering with a list, you will be able to avoid the middle aisles where the processed and high-carb, high-sugar foods are all kept. This will keep you away from temptations and away from foods that you are not going to be eating on this diet.

- **Enter With a List**

One of the most major things to keep in mind when grocery shopping for a new diet is to enter with a list. By doing this, you are going to give yourself a guide and this will prevent you from picking up whatever you crave or whatever you feel like eating at that moment. If you treat it like a treasure hunt, you will be able to cross things off of the list one at a time without venturing to the parts of the grocery store that you do not need to go in and that will simply prove to be a challenge for you to avoid.

- **Choose Vegetables and Other Foods That You Like**

Since the main things that you need to keep in mind are that you should stick to mostly plant-based foods and meals and limit your consumption of fast-foods and packaged snacks, you can allow yourself some room for creativity within your shopping experience. If you prefer broccoli over tomatoes, buy broccoli and find new and fun recipes to use broccoli. If you don't enjoy eggplant, you don't have to eat eggplant at all. By giving yourself some creative freedom within the parameters of your diet, you will be able to let yourself feel like you still have choice and control over what you eat, which will help you stick to the diet and avoid feelings of an uncontrolled life which can lead you to abandon the diet quite quickly.

3 Week WW Weight Loss Plan

To create a weight loss plan for the first three weeks of your new lifestyle, there are two different components. The first is the diet, and the second is exercise. We will begin by looking at what kind of meal plan you can follow, before moving onto the kind of exercise that you can include in your life, whether you are a seasoned exerciser or a newcomer to exercise.

Your Diet

To give you an idea of a common Smart Points allowance on the Weight Watchers Freestyle plan, below I have shared some common examples of Smart Points values associated with several heights, weights, and sex combinations.

1. For a woman who is 5'5, 148 lbs, and 26 years of age, she will get 23 Smart Points daily and 35 Smart Points weekly.
2. For a woman who is 5'2, 130 lbs, and 21 years of age, she will also get 23 Smart Points daily and 35 Smart Points weekly.
3. For a man who is 5'7, 180 lbs, and 35 years of age, he will get 25 Smart Points daily and 42 Smart Points weekly.
4. For a man who is 5'7, 215 lbs, and 52 years of age, he will get 28 Smart Points daily and 42 Smart Points weekly.
5. For a woman who is 5'6, 200 lbs, and 38 years of age, she will get 23 Smart Points daily and 42 Smart Points weekly.

Notice that there is both a daily and a weekly Smart Points value. This is because the weekly value is taking into account the extra Smart Points that are given to provide flexibility over the course of the week for things like special occasions or dinners at a restaurant.

Sample 3-Week Meal Plan

In the chart below, you can see a sample one-week meal plan. For the first week, it will be beneficial for you to follow this meal plan specifically. If you are a vegetarian, you can substitute some of the meals for vegetarian-friendly dishes, but several of the dishes in the chart are vegetarian already.

For your second and third weeks, you can choose one of three options;

1. You can stick with the same weekly meal plan if you are a person who likes and appreciates routine, and you have come to enjoy having your meals planned for you like this.
2. You can substitute the meals that you did not enjoy for new ones, taking them from the cookbook at the end of this book, and keep the meals that you did enjoy the same.
3. You can change up the meal plan entirely, taking them from the cookbook at the end of this book if you are a person who likes to change things up and who does not enjoy eating the same meals each week.

The cookbook that you can find later on in this book is full of tasty and easy to prepare meals, and it also includes the Smart Points values for each of the servings and each of the meals included within. Consult this if you need ideas for meals.

The other thing that you can do is look at the list of Zero Points foods that were listed earlier in this book. By taking ingredients from this list, you can make yourself healthy and quick meals that you will enjoy and that will have the lowest

Smart Points values possible. If you need any more recipes, the Weight Watchers smartphone application and website have a wealth of recipes for you to try that all include the associated Smart Points values.

Day of The Week	Sunday	Monday	Tuesday
Breakfast	Avocado Egg Boats	Smoothie	Non-Fat yogurt with berries
Lunch	Roasted Brussels Sprouts	Ground turkey and vegetable soup	Leftover Vegetarian chili
Dinner	Lamb and Salad	Vegetarian Chili	Pork Chop and Salad
Snacks and Desserts	Brownie	Green Smoothie Snack	Brownie

Wednesday	Thursday	Friday	Saturday
Overnight Oats	Greek Yogurt with blueberries	Smoothie	Spinach Scrambled Eggs
Cauliflower Kale Soup	Leftover Roasted Tomato Soup	Chicken Cacciatore	Grilled Shrimp Kebabs- 0 Points
Roasted Tomato Soup	Broccoli Beef Stir-Fry	Green Beans and Tofu Stir-Fry	Seafood Linguine
Mini Chocolate Chip Cookie	Stone Fruit snack- a peach for example	Grilled Asparagus Snack	Greek Yogurt with Berries

Some other foods that you can substitute this meal plan with include the following,

- Barbacoa beef on rice with black beans and fresh pico de gallo
- Pulled pork lettuce wraps
- Chicken and dumplings
- Split pea soup with ham
- Mushroom soup
- Chicken Cacciatore
- Spaghetti And meat sauce

The recipes for all of the ideas above can be found in the recipe chapter later on in this book, as well as in the chapter on slow cooker and instant pot recipes. If you prefer any of these over the meal ideas included in the chart above, you can instead substitute this. The best thing about it is that you can also take leftovers for lunch at work the next day if you make something for dinner that you just can't get enough of!

Exercise

Exercise is a greatly effective way to lose weight when combined with a healthy eating regimen. If we think about weight loss, we think about exercising because aside from it being a healthy way to strip off unwanted weight, it helps us tone the areas that may have extra skin when we start losing weight.

It is necessary to discuss exercise when discussing weight loss and a diet plan, and in this chapter, we will look at the role exercise should play in your new lifestyle and on your journey to weight loss and improved health, including a decreased risk of disease. Exercising will help you take your mind off of those nagging cravings and will give you a clearer mind overall with which you can look deep inside at those cravings and the emotional issues that are causing them. Exercise will help in all aspects of your life.

Whether you are a seasoned exerciser or someone who has never exercised before in your life, there is an exercise routine out there for you. Do not be discouraged by your experience level when it comes to exercise, as everyone can benefit from it, and everyone must start somewhere. Below, I have given you several ideas for exercise, no matter the experience level you bring with you.

To begin, I will spend some time explaining the different types of exercise and the benefits of each of them, so that you will have a better idea of which types of exercise are best for you and what benefits each of them can provide your body.

Cardiovascular Exercise

Cardiovascular exercise is the type of exercise that involves an elevated heart rate due to activities such as running, riding a bicycle, or swimming. This type of exercise is often referred to as "cardio." This type of exercise is usually done for an extended period of time at a steady state.

When we engage in cardiovascular exercise, our heart rate increases. What this does is carry more oxygen to our muscles so that they can keep exercising. It also carries more oxygen to our brains. More oxygen and blood flow to the brain means that your brain will work more efficiently, more sharply and with more clarity after you finish exercising. More blood flow to the brain also means that it will be generally healthier.

41

Exercising often and for a continued period of time helps to keep the brain structures themselves healthy and in working order. This helps with memory, decision making and learning. Exercise has been shown to be the most effective antidepressant. Many pills are prescribed to treat and beat depression, but the most effective and most natural way to continually boost your mood and to keep it up is through exercise. The effects that exercise has on the brain are far-reaching and numerous.

Resistance Training

Resistance training is a type of exercise that involves using weighs to build up your muscles by doing things like squats, push ups, bicep curls, and so on. This is the type of exercise that you would often do if you go to a gym to exercise. Contrary to popular belief, this type of exercise will not make you bulky and muscular, especially if you are a woman. Instead, it will give you more tone and a leaner body.

When we exercise, we become stronger, faster, and more agile. This not only helps us to exercise better but it helps us in our everyday lives. Moving through life with more ease than before is a great feeling that can only be achieved through exercise. Our bodies are built to move, and they love it when we do move! Our bodies are built to continually become stronger with the more we do, and this is what inevitably happens as soon as we begin exercising regularly.

You can begin to see aesthetic changes as well. You can see your muscles growing, your body toning, and your fat disappearing. These changes on the inside and the outside make us feel great about the body we live in and about the progress we are making mentally.

Taking the time to exercise and to stick with an exercise regime shows our body that we are willing to do the hard work that exercising takes, and it also shows our mind the same thing.

Other Types of Exercise

There are numerous other exercises that do not fit into one of the two categories as described above. These include exercises such as yoga, Pilates, high intensity interval training, group training classes, and so on. While some of these are not considered to be traditional methods of exercise, and others combine both cardiovascular exercise and resistance training exercise, they are no less valid than resistance training or cardiovascular exercise. Many people who are not too enthused about exercise wish to pursue methods that incorporate more of a social aspect, or those that are slower in their movements. If this is what you prefer, this is just as valid as going for a run, as long as you continue to challenge yourself and push your body to try new movements and get that heart rate up!

There are even more ways to be active such as pursuing activities like gardening, dancing, hiking, kayaking and so on. Any activity that gets your heart rate raised and that brings you a sense of joy and accomplishment can be used as an exercise in combination with a diet change in order to bring you weight loss results! When you enjoy the exercises that you are taking part in, you are much more likely to choose to engage in them more often, and much less likely to find excuses to avoid them. By enjoying what you are doing, it will feel like a reward and not like a punishment. For this reason, be sure to choose a form of exercise (or multiple forms) that you enjoy.

3-Week Exercise Plan

In order to begin incorporating exercise into your life, you will need to start out slowly so that you are setting yourself up for the most success possible. If you begin too aggressively, you may become burnt out too soon, leading you to fall off track. Instead, it is best if you ease yourself into your new exercise plan, especially if you do not have much experience exercising, or if you have not been exercising regularly for some time. Below, I have created an exercise plan that will work for you, no matter your experience level. If you have had experience with exercise in the past, but it has been some time since you have participated in a regular exercise regime, choose your category based on your current exercise level so that you can ease into it. If it proves to be much too easy after the initial three weeks, then you can move up in category and challenge yourself a little more. I encourage you to stick with the same plan for the first three weeks however, as this will be enough time for you to get a good sense of how your body is adapting before making any changes. You do not want to make too many changes early on, so stick with whatever you begin with for the first three weeks and then re-evaluate.

If You Are Currently... Sedentary

If you normally don't do much exercise or much walking around, begin by taking the stairs sometimes. Begin also by deciding to walk some places, like to the store down the street or if there is nothing like that around, do some walking around your block. Beginning with this type of movement will get your body used to moving again and will get your muscles and joints moving smoothly.

For the first three weeks, try choosing the stairs and walk to the mailbox or around the block after dinner or before work, or even on your lunch break. By incorporating more movement in your life, this will prepare your body to take on more exercise in the near future. If you are not able to take a walk every day, try to at least incorporate more movement into your daily activities. If you take your child to soccer practice, try walking some laps around the field while they are playing. If you work in an office, stand up and walk around your office once per hour, for example. Try to find areas where you can include even a little bit of movement in order to get started. You do not have to become an Olympic athlete or even any type of athlete overnight, so be gentle with yourself; this new lifestyle will take some getting used to.

If You Are Currently... An Occasional Mover

If you walk occasionally like to a bus stop or to the store on your lunch break, you can begin with a little bit more exercise than someone who is sedentary. Since your muscles and joints are likely somewhat used to being in a standing position, you can begin to jog a little bit. You can jog after dinner around the block a few times, or jog to the store and walk back every few days. You could also take a yoga class if you wish or do some video-guided yoga at home.

For the first three weeks, challenge yourself to go for a jog around the block once every other day. Your body will enjoy this movement that is a little more intense than your usual movements, and it will get your body ready for more intense running or exercise in the future. If you can successfully take yourself for a jog every other day, this will help you to build a great foundation while also helping your body to burn off

45

some extra energy it may have, leading you to a caloric deficit (like we discussed in the first chapter).

If You Are Currently... A Moderate Walker/ A Casual Mover

If you have a moderate level of walking included in your life and you occasionally speed that up to a jog, you can begin to move your body around in new and different ways. Try doing some sit-ups and push-ups at home before or after your run or run to the park and use the playground equipment to do some chin-ups, some two-foot jumps onto a step or run up and down the steps a few times. This will keep your heart rate up and teach your body new ways of moving while allowing your upper body muscles to get a bit of attention as well.

For the first three weeks, challenge yourself to complete a full-body exercise at least three times per week. This exercise will look something like the following,

- Jog to the park
- 10 push-ups
- 20 sit-ups
- 15 box jumps
  Stand in front of a step, ledge, or box that is just below knee-height. Jump up with both feet and land on the box with both feet. Step down one foot at a time. Repeat.
- 20 high knees (each leg)
  Jog on the spot, lifting your knees up as high as you can with each step.
- Jog home

You will first jog or run to a park that is a far enough distance from your house that the run will get your heart pumping. Once you get to the park, you will then complete the exercises as listed and described above. You can do this circuit one time through. After your body becomes very comfortable with this, you can then begin to increase the number of repetitions of each exercise, or you can repeat the entire cycle multiple times over. This circuit is very versatile as there are many factors that you can change in order to continue challenging yourself for quite a while in order to avoid a plateau!

On the other days of the week, try to go for a light jog around the block or a walk around the neighborhood.

If You Are Currently... A Casual Mover/ A Moderate Runner

If you run frequently and have some bodyweight exercise sessions every now and again, try visiting a gym and doing some exercises with some more weight. You can try squatting, pressing some things overhead, and maybe some bicep curls. This will challenge your muscles in ways that your own body weight cannot and take you to a new level of fitness and mood-boosting.

Challenge yourself for the initial three weeks to visit the gym at least 2-3 times per week. In the gym, you can use some light dumbbells to do things like shoulder press, bicep curls, chest press, and squats. All of these can be found online, and you can feel free to switch them out for any other simple exercises as you wish. Ensure you begin with light weights and ask the gym staff for assistance if you need it- safety is the number one priority!

On the other days, go for a run or a bike ride outside or on a treadmill or stationary bike. You can also include some bodyweight exercises on these days if you are not too sore from your gym sessions.

If You Are Currently... An Experienced Runner

If you are an experienced runner, you are likely quite familiar with the feeling of runner's high. You are likely quite familiar with how exercise can change your mood around and take you from feeling hopeless to hopeful. If you want to try some new forms of exercise, try adding in a regular routine in the gym lifting weights. This will take your running to new heights and will give you a new type of exercise experience to break up the running days.

For the first three weeks of this program in particular, you can try to go for a run every day. If there is one day that you can get into a gym and do some simple exercises after your run, that will help you to burn the most calories possible. One other day per week, either before or after you daily run, do some exercises such as push-ups, bodyweight squats, sit-ups, pull-ups, and any other exercises you wish to do using your bodyweight.

If You Are Currently... An Experienced Exerciser

If you are experienced when it comes to exercise, good for you! Continue to challenge yourself in new ways and teach your body new ways of moving. Exercise does nothing but good things, so keep up your routine.

You can look over all of the above categories and come up with an exercise plan that best fits your area of expertise in terms of exercise, as well as a plan that includes some type of exercise every day. For example, you can design a plan, such as the plan I have laid out for you below. This is an example, but feel free to use this exact one, or to substitute some of the sections below with different choices. You can continue to follow this plan for the first three weeks and then evaluate the plan to see what works for you and what doesn't. Continue to try to include exercise each day!

Day	Monday	Tuesday	Wednesday
Exercise Plan	3 Kilometer Run, followed by 5 sets of the following: 20 push-ups, 20 sit-ups, 20 pull-ups.	15km Bike ride with 3x sprint efforts of 30 seconds each.	Weight Room Workout: Squats holding weights Bench Press or Chest Press Lunges holding weights

Thursday	Friday	Saturday	Sunday
5 Kilometer Run	Bodyweight workout Push-ups, Sit-ups, ab exercises, jumping exercises.	3 Kilometer Run, followed by 5 sets of the following: 20 push-ups, 20 sit-ups, 20 pull-ups.	Leisurely walk or jog for fun and enjoyment.

If You Are Currently... A Woman Over the Age of 50

Since exercising helps women to regain some of the muscle mass lost due to age, it can be greatly beneficial for women to exercise into their older years. It is important to be aware of how to do this safely though. It can be safer to stick to low-impact exercises, so exercises that avoid jumping or any sort of quick, jarring movements. Instead, spending some time on an exercise bike (or a real bike) or elliptical machine can be good as they reduce impact and are therefore better for a woman's joints. Things like running involve more impact, so if you have joint pain, it is best to avoid this type of exercise. Further, lifting some small weights or walking with weights in your hands can help you to build back some muscle, which will lead to an increase in your resting rate of metabolism (the number of calories your body burns when it is just sitting, at rest in order to execute living functions such as breathing or sitting) . Your overall health will be greatly improved by the increase in muscle, the improvement of your joint health and the lowered risk of diseases such as heart disease (which is reduced by doing aerobic exercise). Staying active in your 50's is a great decision and every woman who is capable should add exercise into their lives, regardless of the diet that they follow.

For any level of exerciser or mover, challenging your body in new ways will be beneficial in so many aspects of your life. In addition to its effects on the brain, body, and mood, it will help with your health in the long-run and the ease with which you will be able to complete everyday tasks like climbing the stairs and throwing a ball to your child. The goal is to make this a part of the new lifestyle we are working towards which will make it so ingrained in your life that you will not want to go without.

After the Initial Three Weeks: Exercise

After the initial three weeks, you can then evaluate yourself again and see how your body is feeling. If you were sedentary before beginning, and you have successfully taken a walk each night after dinner, for example, you can now call yourself an occasional mover. From here, you can then take on the exercise plan included in the occasional mover section instead. If after the first three weeks, you did not move as much as you wanted to, stick with the same plan for some more time and continue trying to challenge yourself by trying to make movement a regular part of your life!

When we exercise, our brain releases chemicals that tell us that we enjoy the effects that the exercise is giving us. This feeling is known as "runner's high," and it is that elation you feel after you run a long distance or complete a workout. When you are feeling down and you exercise, your mood will lift because of this runner's high. For this reason, it is not so important what kind of physical exercise you do, but rather the fact that you engage in it regularly in order to help you feel motivated and to keep your mood positive. This runner's high can be compared to those rewarded feelings that the highly sugary foods give us, but with runner's high, the feeling of elation and accomplishment last way longer than the rewarded happy feelings we get from eating food. Sugary or salty fast foods make our brains feel happy, but our body feels heavy and lethargic. Exercise, as I mentioned, makes all of our body parts feel great at the same time, and this is why the effects of runner's high are so long-lasting. For this reason, choose something you enjoy doing and you will not have to force yourself to exercise, you will simply want to engage in those activities!

Chapter 4: WW Freestyle Cookbook

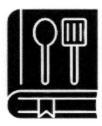

In this chapter, you will find the WW Freestyle cookbook that you have been waiting for! This cookbook includes recipes for any and every kind of food that you could hope for! If after reading the previous three chapters, you are feeling a little overwhelmed, don't worry! That is completely normal. This cookbook includes a variety of recipes including breakfast, lunch, dinner, dessert, snack and protein recipes including their Smart Points values! With this cookbook, you will never be without a recipe for any occasion and this will help you on those challenging days when you just aren't sure of what to make for dinner. Instead of turning to takeout, take out this book and you will have a healthy, delicious dinner that also fits within your Smart Points in no time!

Power Breakfast Recipes

We are going to begin with the first meal of the day- breakfast! This section includes delicious recipes for breakfast, both of the sweet and the savory variety.

Avocado Egg Bowls

Smart Points Value: 3 Points Per Serving

NUTRITIONAL INFORMATION:
Serving size 130g (One half of recipe)
Calories 215
Calories from fat 163
Fat 18g
Carbohydrates 8g
Fiber 2.6g
Protein 9g

INGREDIENTS:
- Coconut oil- 1 Teaspoon
- Organic, free-range eggs-2
- Salt and pepper- to sprinkle
- Large & ripe avocado- 1

For Garnishing:
- Chopped walnuts, as many as you like
- Fresh thyme
- Balsamic reduction

INSTRUCTIONS:
1. Slice your avocado into halves.
2. Scoop out a little bit of the flesh enough so that the egg can fit inside
3. Slice off a small section of the skin on the bottom so it will sit flat when you set it down.
4. Open the eggs and put each of the yolks into a small bowl or glass

5. Combine the egg whites together in one bowl. To taste, sprinkle pepper/salt.
6. Warm your coconut oil using a pan with a lid on top of medium to high heat. Add the avocadoes with the green side down.
7. Cook them for about 30 seconds, or until they become slightly golden in color
8. Turn over the avocados and pour in the egg whites. Lower the heat, put the lid on top, and cook the egg whites in the avocado boats for 15-20 minutes or until the egg whites are cooked.
9. Then, gently add the yolks into the egg whites and continue to cook for 3-5 more minutes or until the yolks have cooked until the level you want them.
10. Pass them over to a serving plate and top them with walnuts, thyme, and the balsamic reduction, if you wish.

Breakfast Drinks and Frozen Dessert Recipes

Healthy Snack Smoothie

Smart Points Value: 0 Smart Points

NUTRITIONAL INFORMATION:
Calories: 117
Fat: 15g
Protein: 20g
Carbohydrates: 5g

Preparation Time: 5 Minutes
Cook Time: 1 Minute
Total Time: 6 Minutes
Yield: 1 serving

INGREDIENTS:
- 1 ¼ cups water
- ½ cup kale or spinach, or both (¼ Cup each) if you prefer
- ½ avocado, sliced into smaller pieces
- ¾ cup cucumber, sliced into smaller pieces
- 1 cup green grapes
- ¼ teaspoon ginger, peeled and grated
- 1 banana
- Honey to taste

DIRECTIONS:

1. Add all of these ingredients into your blender, in the order they appear above.
2. Blend them until the mixture is smooth
3. Taste it!

Pour into a glass and serve

Coconut Blueberry Smoothie

Smart Points Value: 4 Smart Points

NUTRITIONAL INFORMATION:
Calories: 215
Fat 10g
Carbohydrates: 7g
Fiber 3g
Protein 23g

Preparation Time: 5 Minutes
Cook Time: 1 Minute
Total Time: 6 Minutes
Yield:1 serving

INGREDIENTS:
- Coconut or almond milk, unsweetened- 1 cup
- Blueberries- 1 cup
- Vanilla extract- 1tsp
- Coconut oil- 1 teaspoon

DIRECTIONS:
1. Add all of these ingredients into your blender in the order they appear above.
2. Blend them until the mixture is smooth
3. Taste it and add as much honey as you desire

Pour into a glass and serve

Salad Recipes

This section includes salad recipes that are not only full of necessary vitamins and minerals, but they will also fit within your Smart Points allowance with ease!

Caprese Salad With Beets and Avocado

Smart Points Value: 4 Points Per Serving

NUTRITIONAL INFORMATION:
Serving Size (1/2 recipe)
Calories: 444
Total Carbohydrates: 5g
Fiber: 1g
Net Carbohydrates: 4g
Fat: 38g
Protein: 22g

INGREDIENTS:
- Unsalted almonds, raw and chopped - ¼ cup
- Kale- 100 grams
- Fresh basil, thinly sliced- to garnish
- Minced shallots- 1 tablespoon
- Buffalo mozzarella cheese, sliced- 1 cup
- Beet- 1 small
- Sea salt- ¼ teaspoon
- Balsamic vinegar- 2 tablespoons
- Extra virgin olive oil- 1 tablespoon
- Freshly ground black pepper- as much as desired

INSTRUCTIONS:

1. Preheat the oven to 400 degrees Fahrenheit. Wrap the beet in some foil. Roast the beet in the foil just until it becomes soft enough to put a fork through it, about 1 hour. When the beet is cool enough to handle, peel it, and cut it into about 8 slices.

2. Meanwhile, using a small vessel, whisk to combine the shallots, vinegar, oil, ⅛ teaspoon salt, and ⅛ teaspoon pepper.

3. Arrange your beet, cheese, and kale on 2 plates and sprinkle with nuts and basil. Sprinkle evenly with the remaining salt and pepper, and drizzle evenly with the vinaigrette.

Soup Recipes

On a cold winter night, what is better than soup! If you are wondering what kind of soup will fit with your Weight Watchers Freestyle plan, look no further!

Cauliflower Rice Curry Kale Soup

Smart Points Value: 1 Point Per Serving

NUTRITIONAL INFORMATION:
Serving Size: ¼ of recipe
Fat: 8g
Carbohydrates: 20g
Fiber: 9g
Protein: 6g
Calories: 162

30 minutes: Preparation Time
20 minutes: Cook Time:
55 minutes: Total Time:
4 servings total yield

INGREDIENTS:
- Chopped carrots- 2 cups
- Garlic powder- 1 teaspoon
- Garlic, minced- 1 teaspoon
- Curry powder -2 to 3 tablespoons
- Kale, Without Stems, and chopped-8 leaves
- Salt- to taste
- Olive oil for roasting- 2 or 3 tablespoons

- 1 drained can of white beans of choice
- Broth (chicken or vegetable)- 4 cups
- Red pepper or chili flakes- ½ teaspoon
- Paprika- ½ teaspoon
- Sea salt- ¼ teaspoon
- Cauliflower florets- 6 cups
- Chopped Red onion- 3/4 cup
- Cumin- ½ teaspoon
- Black pepper- ½ teaspoon
- Olive oil or avocado oil- 2 teaspoons

Feel Free to add any other vegetables you wish, or substitute for others that you prefer.

INSTRUCTIONS:
1. Prewarm the oven to 400 degrees Fahrenheit.
2. Get a bowl and combine the cauliflower with your garlic powder, curry powder, paprika, salt, cumin, and three tablespoons of oil.
3. place the tossed cauliflower florets onto a cookie sheet or a pan. Put them in the oven to cook the florets for 20 to 22 mins, or until they are softened but not too well-done. If anything, make sure they are slightly undercooked.
4. Remove them from the oven and put them to the side.
5. Begin to prepare the rest of your vegetables by slicing them accordingly.
6. Put your roasted cauliflower into a blender, and pulse them a couple of times, until the cauliflower gets chopped or "riced." If you do not own a food processor, you can simply cut it into very small pieces. Alternatively, you could buy cauliflower that has already been riced for you and then toss and cook it in the oven.

7. Ensure that you don't overwork your cauliflower in the food processor when it is roasted. You don't it to become a puree; you just want it to be lightly chopped.
8. When the cauliflower is completely riced, also your kale and vegetables are cut up, you can then begin to prepare your cooking pot.
9. Place 2 tsp of oil, the onion, the garlic in big pot. cook this for 6 mins, or until it is aromatic.
10. Next, incorporate the beans, vegetables, broth, cauliflower "rice," red chili pepper, black pepper.
11. Bring this to a boil, and then let it simmer, about 22 mins, until all of the vegetables become softened.
12. Sprinkle some salt, to taste, when it is cooked and ready to serve.
13. Garnish this with herbs and cracker crumbs if you wish.

Roasted Tomato Soup

Smart Points Value: 1 Point Per Serving

NUTRITIONAL INFORMATION:
Calories: 95
Fat: 8g
Total Carbs: 1g
Net Carbs: 1g
Protein: 3g

Serving Size: 1 cup or 1/6 of recipe

Cooking Time: 40 minutes
Preparation Time: 5.5 minutes
Total Time: 45 minutes
Servings: 5-7 servings

INGREDIENTS:
- 6 Leaves Fresh basil (cut into ribbons)
- 1 onion, red. Chopped
- 1/2 tsp Sea salt
- 1 tsp sugar
- 2 carrots, cut into small pieces
- 1/4 tsp Black pepper
- 3 garlic cloves, cut into small pieces
- 1/4 cup Heavy cream (or coconut cream for paleo)
- 10 medium Roma tomato (cut into 1" cubes)
- 4 cloves Garlic (minced)
- 2 tbsp Olive oil
- 2 cup Chicken bone broth (or any chicken broth)

- 1 tbsp Herbs de Provence

INSTRUCTIONS:
1. Preheat your oven to 400 degrees Fahrenheit (or 204 degrees Celsius).
2. Line a baking sheet with some aluminum foil and lightly grease it.
3. Begin with your tomato pieces and toss them in the olive oil as well as the minced garlic. Arrange this on the baking sheet you prepared in a single layer.
4. Pop this into your oven to cook it for approximately 20 or 25 mins, or until your tomato skin begins to pucker up.
5. When ready, move these tomato pieces into a blender along with the oil and liquid as well as the garlic on the baking sheet. Puree all of this in the blender until it becomes smooth. (This will work the best if you use a high-powered blender. If you don't have one, do this in smaller batches using a regular blender. Instead, you could use a blender to blend this inside of this original pot that will be needed next.)
6. Pour your newly blended tomato mixture into a pot and put it on the stove on medium heat. Add in your broth.
7. Season this mixture in the pot with your Herbs de Provence, black pepper, and sea salt as you wish to taste.
8. Let this pot simmer here for about 10 to 15 minutes.
9. Stir in the basil.
10. You are ready to serve and enjoy

Snack Recipes

Snacks don't have to be unhealthy and make you feel guilty as soon as you eat them! In this section you will find healthy snacks that will curb your hunger while keeping you within your Smart Points budget! No longer do snacks have to make you feel guilty and shameful; these snacks are delicious, quick and nutritious.

Grilled Asparagus

Smart Points Value: 1 Smart Point Per Serving

Serving: 4 spears of asparagus
Calories: 50 calories
Carbohydrates: 3.5g,
Protein: 4g,
Fat: 2.5g,
Fiber: 1.5g,

5 mins: prep time
10 mins: cook time
15 mins: total time

INGREDIENTS:
- Olive Oil for greasing
- Kosher salt-for tasting
- black pepper- for tasting
- Asparagus, rimmed at the ends-16
- Parmigiano Reggiano, 1 ounce

INSTRUCTIONS:

1. Drizzle your asparagus on a plate with some olive oil and season it as you wish with black pepper and a pinch of salt.
2. Light up your grill onto only light heat.
3. When the grill is hot enough, clean, and then oil the grates before cooking.
4. Place the asparagus onto your warm grill a begin cooking it for a duration of about 6 mins, with the lid on. Continue cooking them on low heat and turn them every couple of minutes so that they don't burn.
5. Slice the parmigiano very thinly and then add this to the hot asparagus.

Fresh Green Beans With Tofu and Mushroom Stir-Fry

Smart Points Value: 4 Points Per Serving

NUTRITIONAL INFORMATION:
Serving: 1 Serving (1/6 of Recipe)
Calories: 94kcal
Carbohydrates: 9g
Protein: 5g
Fat: 5g
Saturated Fat: 2g
Fiber: 3g
Sugar: 4g

15 minutes: Prep Time
20 minutes: Cook Time
35 minutes: Total Time

Servings: 6 Servings

INGREDIENTS:
- 1/4 teaspoon kosher salt
- 1-pound thin green beans trimmed
- 1 cup tofu, firm variety
- 1 tablespoon minced fresh sage
- 1 large shallot minced
- 12 ounces mushrooms thinly sliced
- 1 teaspoon olive oil
- 3 tablespoons parsley minced

- 1 tablespoon minced fresh thyme leaves
- 1/4 teaspoon freshly ground black pepper
- 1 tablespoon ginger, grated
- 1 tablespoon soy sauce

INSTRUCTIONS:
1. Salt a large saucepan full of water and heat it up until it boils. Mix your beans into water and cook them until they become tender but still a little crispy, this will take approximately 2 minutes. Drain the water and immediately move the cooked beans to a bowl full of ice and water in order to stop them from cooking any further.
2. Drain the beans of the water once again and set them aside.
3. Put your tofu inside of a big frying pan on one half level of heat. heat your tofu until it becomes crispy. Move the tofu to a paper towel and crumble it with your hands before setting it off to the side for later.
4. Put olive oil into the same frying pan you used before and turn it on to medium-high heat. Add in your mushrooms and shallots, and cook them until they are tender, this will take approx. 2 to 3 minutes.
5. Add the green beans to the frying pan again and cook the entire thing for 1 to 2 minutes more, stir it often.
6. Add in the sage, thyme, parsley, pepper and, salt, and stir it to combine. Cook this for another minute, before re-adding your tofu.
7. Serve this dish either hot or at room temperature.

Beef, Pork and Lamb Recipes

Sometimes you need a nice protein to be the star of your dinner. Your family will love it and so will you! Meat won't take up too many of your Smart Points, as you will see in the recipes included in this section.

Beef and Broccoli Stir-Fry

Smart Points Value: 3 Points Per Serving

Preparation Time: 16 minutes
Cooking time: 12 minutes
Total Time: 28 minutes

Makes: 4 Servings
Serving Size: 1 and ¼ of a cup or ¼ of total recipe

INGREDIENTS:
- Sirloin Beef, Lean and thinly sliced- ¾ of a pound
- Cornstarch- 2 and 1/3 tablespoons
- Red pepper flakes- 2 tablespoons
- Chicken Broth, Reduced Sodium- 1 Cup
- Salt- ¼ teaspoon
- Broccoli- 5 cups
- Water- ¼ cup
- Ginger root, minced- 1 tablespoon
- Garlic, minced- 2 tablespoons
- Soy Sauce, low sodium- ¼ cup

INSTRUCTIONS:

1. Take a large plate and spread the cornstarch and the salt around the plate evenly. Take the beef strips and coat them with the mixture.
2. Using a wok or a deep pan, put the oil in and heat it up on medium to high heat level
3. Put the beef in when the pan is hot and cook this until it is cooked all the way through- you will know as it will turn brown. This will take about 4 minutes.
4. Use a slotted spoon and take the beef out of the pan and place it on a new plate.
5. In the same pan with the heated oil and the beef drippings, put ½ cup of reduced-sodium chicken broth. Begin stirring this in the pan to combine everything and loosen the residue on the pan.
6. Put the broccoli in the pan and cook it with the lid on. Add some water if you need.
7. When the broccoli is becoming softer but not fully cooked yet- this will take about 3 minutes, take the lid off and put the garlic, ginger, and red pepper flakes in. Fry this until it becomes noticeably fragrant, which will take roughly one minute.
8. Using a vessel of your choice, mix together the rest of the broth (1/2 cup), the soy sauce, the water, and the rest of the cornstarch (1/2 tablespoon). Stir it to mix well.
9. Put this sauce mix into the wok and stir everything to combine it all together.
10. Bring the heat down to a medium to low level and let this simmer.
11. Simmer for about a minute, until it begins to become thicker.
12. Put the beef in the pan once again and stir everything so the beef becomes coated.
13. It is now ready to serve!

Pork Chops

Smart Points Value: 4 Points Per Serving

NUTRITIONAL INFORMATION:

Calories: 308
Fat: 18 grams
Carbohydrates: 4 grams
Protein: 30 grams

Preparation time: 10 minutes
Cooking time: 10 minutes
Total time: 20 minutes

INGREDIENTS:
- Lean Pork- 1 lb in 4 ounce pieces
- Salt- ¾ of a teaspoon
- Lime Juice- 6 Tablespoons
- Black Pepper- ¼ of a teaspoon
- Garlic- 1 and ½ teaspoon minced
- Red Onion- 1 small, chopped
- Cilantro, Chopped- 2 tablespoons
- Extra Virgin Olive Oil- 2 teaspoons
- Oregano and Cumin, Dried- 1 teaspoon each

INSTRUCTIONS:
1. Take a medium bowl and mix together the onion, 3 tablespoons of the lime juice, ¼ teaspoon of salt and the cilantro.
2. Allow this mixture to wilt the cilantro by letting it sit for some time. You may stir or toss it every now and

then. You can let it sit in the fridge, or at room temperature.

3. Take a food storage bag and put the pork chops, the rest of the salt and lime juice, the pepper, olive oil, garlic, cumin, and the oregano. Mix this around in the bag so that it is combined, and the lamb is coated.
4. Let this marinate for about two hours in the fridge.
5. Take a pan and moisten it so that the lamb will not stick to it. You can use a cooking spray or some oil.
6. Put the pork on the pan and let it cook. Test the temperature to check the cook and ensure that it reaches a temperature of 145 degrees at the thickest part of the meat. This will take about 9 minutes.
7. Remove from heat and put your wilted onion and cilantro mix on top for garnish.

Roasted Leg of Lamb

Smart Points Value: 4 Points Per Serving

Preparation time: 10 minutes
Cooking time: 1 hour and 30 minutes
Total Time: 1 hour and 40 minutes

Makes: 8 Servings
Serving Size: 2 Slices of Lamb

INGREDIENTS:
- Lamb legs, Boneless, Tied and Rolled Up- 3 and a half pounds
- Lemon Zest- 1 tablespoon
- Garlic- 3 Full Bulbs
- Thyme, Fresh, Chopped- 2 tablespoons
- Salt, Kosher- To taste
- Pepper, Black- ½ teaspoon ground
- Olive oil- 3 tablespoons

INSTRUCTIONS:
1. First, start by preheating your oven to 375 degrees Fahrenheit.
2. Take a roasting pan and put aluminum foil in the bottom of it.
3. Take 4 cloves of garlic and mine them so they are fine. In a small bowl, mix this garlic with the lemon zest, salt, and pepper, 2 tablespoons of olive oil and the thyme. Mix this together.
4. Using your olive oil mixture, rub it over your lamb.
5. Put the lamb legs in the roasting pan lined with foil.

6. Using the rest of the garlic, peel it and dip it in the rest of your olive oil. Then, spread the garlic cloves and the oil around the lamb in the pan.
7. Put this in the oven and cook until it is medium rare. Using a thermometer, test and ensure that it is 145 degrees Fahrenheit. This will take about 75 minutes.
8. Take the lamb out and put it on a cutting board so that it can rest for 15 minutes.
9. Check the roasting pan to see if the garlic has softened. If not, put the pan with garlic back in the oven and let this roast for 10 more minutes.
10. Cut your lamb into pieces of about ¼ of an inch in thickness.
11. Take the garlic from the pan and squeeze the garlic and oil on the slices of lamb.
12. Using the fat juices left in the pan, drizzle it over the lamb.
13. Serve!

Seafood Recipes

Seafood is a great choice any time of year! What's more, many vegetarians choose to include seafood as their main source of protein. In this section, I will share a delicious seafood recipe for you to try.

Seafood Linguine

Smart Points Value: 7 Points Per Serving

Total Time: 40 minutes
Makes: Serves 4
Serving Size: ¼ of recipe

INGREDIENTS:
- Scallions, sliced- 8
- Linguine, Cooked- 4 Cups
- Salt- ¼ teaspoon
- Dry White Wine- 2 tablespoons
- Garlic, Minced- 3 cloves
- Extra virgin olive oil- 1 tablespoon
- Shrimp, Peeled and Cooked- ½ pound
- Crab Meat, Cooked and Flaked-1/2 pound
- Red pepper flakes- ¼ teaspoon
- Thyme Leaves, dried- ¼ teaspoon
- Lemon Juice, Fresh- 1 tablespoon

INSTRUCTIONS:
1. Ensure that your crab meat and your shrimp are cooked and ready to be eaten!

2. Cook the dry pasta using the method specified on the container.
3. Heat up the oil in a large size pan
4. Put in the garlic and the scallions, and then cook this until it is softened. This will take about 3 minutes.
5. Once softened, add in the crab and shrimp, as well as the lemon juice, salt, white wine, thyme, and red pepper flakes. Stir continuously and let this heat thoroughly. This will take approximately three minutes.
6. Put the cooked linguine on a plate and then top it with your seafood and scallion mixture.

¼ of recipe is one serving size.

Enjoy!

Vegetarian Recipes

Vegetarians can also benefit from this cookbook and find delicious, Smart Points-friendly meals to make for lunch or dinner!

Roasted Brussels Sprouts With Pecans and Maple Glaze

Smart Points Value: 4 Points Per Serving

Yields: 4 servings
12 mins: preparation time
38 mins: cook time
50 mins: total time

INGREDIENTS:
- Brussels Sprouts, fresh- 1 pound
- Pecans, chopped- ¼ cup
- Olive oil- 1 tablespoon
- extra olive oil to oil the baking tray
- Pepper and salt for tasting
- Balsamic Vinegar- 3 tablespoons
- Maple Syrup- 2 Tablespoons

INSTRUCTIONS:
1. Warm the oven to 350 degrees Fahrenheit or 175 Celcius.
2. Rub a large pan or any vessel you wish to use with a little bit of olive oil; you can use a paper towel or a pastry brush.

3. Cut off the ends of the Brussels Sprouts if you need to and then cut then in a lengthwise direction into halves. (fear not if a few of the leaves come off of them, some may become deliciously crunchy during cooking)
4. Chop up all of the pecans using a knife and then measure them for the amount as specified.
5. Put your Brussels Sprouts as well as the sliced pecans inside a mixing container, then cover the entire thing with some olive oil, pepper as well as salt (be generous).
6. Arrange all of your pecans and Brussels Sprouts onto your roasting pan without overlapping them at all.
7. Let this cook for 30 to 35 mins, or when they become tender and can be pierced with a fork easily. Stir during cooking if you wish to get a more even browning.
8. Combine the balsamic, the maple syrup, and ¼ teaspoon of salt. Put this in a pot and on the stove for
9. Serve them hot.

Vegan Recipes

Vegans are those who choose not to eat any animal products, including eggs, dairy and meat. In this section, I will share with you some delicious vegan recipes that are great for your Weight Watchers Freestyle diet plan.

Vegan Artichoke Dip

Smart Points Value: 1 Point Per Serving

NUTRITIONAL INFORMATION:
Calories: 63
Carbohydrates: 3 grams
Protein: 1g
Fat: 0g
Calories from fat: 1

Makes 4 Servings

INGREDIENTS:
- Artichoke Hearts, Canned- 14 ounces
- Salt- ½ of a teaspoon
- Balsamic Vinegar- 1teaspoon
- Pepper- ¼ of a teaspoon
- Cumin- ½ of a teaspoon
- Garlic- 1 Clove

INSTRUCTIONS:
1. Pour the water out of the artichokes, but keep one half of a cup of the liquid for later.
2. Combine these items using a food processor or blender and mix them until they are thoroughly mixed together.
3. If the mixture is thicker than you like, add the liquid from the can of artichokes and mix it into the dip using the blender once again. Add it only a Tbsp at a time so that you don't make it too runny and so that it mixes well.
4. Taste it and add more seasoning if need be.
5. Put it in a bowl and serve it!

Vegan Chana Masala

Smart Points Value: 1 Smart Point Per Serving

NUTRITIONAL INFORMATION:
Calories: 371
Calories from Fat: 88
Total Fat: 10g
Carbohydrates: 59 grams
Protein: 17 grams

Servings: Makes 4 Servings

INGREDIENTS:
- Olive Oil-1 Tablespoon
- Cayenne Pepper- 1/8 of a tablespoon
- Diced Tomatoes- 28 ounces diced
- Garam Masala- 2 tablespoons
- Jalapeno Pepper- 1
- Onion- 1 diced
- Ginger- 1 tablespoon shaved
- Garlic- 4 Cloves minced
- Chickpeas- canned- 28 ounces (be sure to drain the liquid and rinse them before using them in the recipe)

INSTRUCTIONS:
1. Take a big wok and put the olive oil into it
2. Once heated, add in your onions and sauté them until they are sweating and softened. This will take about 5 minutes.
3. Add in your ginger, jalapeno, and your garlic, and then cook this mixture for another minute

4. Sprinkle in your spices (pepper, salt, coriander, turmeric, garam masala, cumin, cayenne pepper). Then, cook this for another minute. The mixture will become fragrant as you do this.
5. Add your chickpeas and tomatoes into the fragrant mixture in the wok. Let this simmer.
6. Cover the pan and let this simmer for about twenty minutes.
7. After it simmers for the allotted time, give it a taste test and season it if you feel it could be spicier or if it needs more salt. You might want to mix in some more of the garam masala if you want it to be stronger in flavor.
8. Serve and enjoy this meal that is only 1 Smart Point per serving!

Pasta and Grain Recipes

Who doesn't love pasta? Pasta is a staple in many households, and just because you are following a Weight Watchers Freestyle diet now does not mean that you cannot enjoy pasta anymore. In this section, I will share with you a delicious recipe for your next pasta night.

Stovetop Macaroni And Cheese

Smart Points Value: 9 Points Per Serving

NUTRITIONAL INFORMATION:
Calories: 322
Calories From Fat: 90
Fat: 10 grams
Fiber: 2 grams
Carbohydrates: 39 grams
Protein: 22 grams

Makes: 8 Servings
Serving Size: ¾ of a cup

INGREDIENTS:
- Elbow Macaroni- 2 and a half cups, uncooked
- Salt- 1 teaspoon
- Light Cream Cheese- ¼ of a cup
- Pepper- ¼ teaspoon
- Flour, All-purpose- 4 tablespoons
- Dry Mustard- 2 teaspoons
- Cayenne Pepper- ¼ of a teaspoon
- Milk, Fat-Free- 2 and ¼ cups

- Sharp Cheddar, Reduced Fat- 2 and ½ cups

INSTRUCTIONS:
1. To start, cook the macaroni just like the bag tells you to. Then, pour off the water and put this off to the side
2. While you are waiting for your macaroni to cook, you can begin to make the sauce. In a bowl, whisk together the salt and pepper, the dry mustard, the flour, and the cayenne pepper. Then, transfer this to a saucepan and add the milk. Whisk this in order to combine it.
3. Simmer the mixture and add in the cream cheese one teaspoon at a time so that it mixes well.
4. Bring this saucepan of ingredients to a boil by putting the pot onto medium to high power level, and make sure that you whisk the entire time.
5. Once it boils, bring the heat down to a simmer and let it bubble, stirring this every now and then until the cream cheese becomes melted and the sauce gets thicker.
6. Take the sauce off of the heat and drop the sharp cheddar into the cheese sauce. Stir this until it is melted and mixed throughout.
7. Put the cooked macaroni into the pot with the cheese sauce and mix this around until all of the pasta is covered in cheese sauce.
8. Season with more salt and pepper if you wish and serve in ¾ cup servings.

Breads, Cookies and Cake Recipes

Just like Weight Watchers Freestyle does not make you give up pasta, it also does not make you give up cookies or other sweets. In this section, you will find recipes for these sweets that won't use up your entire daily or weekly Smart Points budget!

Weight Watchers Brownies

Smart Points Value: 3 Points Per Serving

NUTRITIONAL INFORMATION:
Calories: 107
Calories from fat: 90
Fat: 10g
Carbohydrates: 5.7g
Fiber: 2.9g
Protein: 2.5g

10 minutes: Prep Time
20 minutes: Cook Time
30 minutes: Total Time
Serving- serves 16 People
Serving Size- 1/16 or recipe

INGREDIENTS:
- Plain, Low-fat Yogurt- ½ of a cup
- Sugar- ¾ of a cup
- Cocoa Powder, Unsweetened- ¾ of a cup
- Flour, all-purpose- ½ of a cup

- Baking Powder- ½ of a teaspoon
- Baking soda- ½ teaspoon
- Sea salt- ¼ teaspoon
- Vanilla extract- 2 tablespoons

INSTRUCTIONS:
1. Preheat your oven to 350 degrees and line an 8x8 inch pan with parchment paper, leaving some sticking up to use as a handle to get the brownies out of the pan.
2. In a medium bowl, add in the sugar, the cocoa, the salt, and the flour. Beat these together using an electric hand mixer. Then, add vanilla and yogurt and combine it all using your hands.
3. Put the batter in the pan and spread it around, so it is even at all corners.
4. Put it into the oven and bake it until the edges just begin to darken, the center rises a little bit, and a toothpick inserted in the center comes out clean, about 20-21 minutes. Do NOT over bake!
5. Let cool in the pan for 20 minutes and then gently use the parchment paper handles to lift the brownies onto a wire rack to cool COMPLETELY.
6. Once totally cooled, slice, and DEVOUR!

Chocolate Chip Cookies

Smart Points Value: 1 Smart Point Per Serving

NUTRITIONAL INFORMATION:
Serving Size: 1 Cookie
Recipe Makes: 48 Mini Cookies

Calories: 100
Fat: 5g
Carbohydrates: 16 grams
Protein: 0.5 grams

INGREDIENTS:
- Butter, Salted- 2 Tablespoons
- Flour, All-Purpose- ¼ of a cup
- Dark Brown Sugar, Packed- ½ of a cup
- Egg White- 1
- Chocolate Chips, Semi-Sweet- ½ of a cup
- Salt- 1/8 of a teaspoon
- Canola oil- 2 tablespoons
- Vanilla Extract- 1 Tablespoon
- Baking Soda- ¼ of a teaspoon

INSTRUCTIONS:
1. Begin by preheating your oven to 375 degrees Fahrenheit or 190 degrees Celsius
2. Take a bowl and put your butter, sugar, and oil into it. Then mix them together.
3. Add the vanilla, the egg white, and the salt into the same bowl as the butter mixture and then mix them all to combine it well.

87

4. Take another bowl and put in the baking soda and the flour, and then mix this into the original batter mix.
5. Stir in your chocolate chips until they are mixed throughout
6. Now comes the time to put them on the pan. For each serving, spoon out one half of a teaspoon of batter and put it onto a baking sheet. Make sure there is space between the cookies as they will spread out as they cook.
7. Bake these for about 5 minutes, or until you notice that the edges are becoming browned.
8. Remove them from the oven and let them sit to cool down for twenty minutes.

The recipes in this section are meant to bring you joy in the kitchen and with your family, and to show you that you do not have to give up on enjoying the foods you love just because you are looking to lose weight and lead a healthier lifestyle. I hope you enjoy making some of these foods and sharing them with your loved ones!

BONUS! Turkey Dinner Recipe

Are you afraid that you have to miss out on your traditional turkey dinner this thanksgiving because you are following a new diet?

Think again!

Smart Points Value:
2 Smart Points Per 2-Ounce Slice of Turkey (White meat with skin or without, dark meat with no skin)
3 Smart Points Per 2- Ounce Slice of Dark Meat with Skin On
Bacon, One Slice- 1 Point

According to the Smart Points values above, you can eat the turkey dinner below as long as you are looking at the number of slices of turkey and the amount of skin that you are eating as well. Keeping track of this will ensure that you are not falling off track by participating in traditional festive eating!

NUTRITIONAL INFORMATION:
Serving size: 12g

1 hour: Prep Time
30 Minutes: Cook Time
1 hour, 30 minutes: Total Time

Servings: Makes 12 Servings

INGREDIENTS:
- Turkey, including bones- 20lbs, 1 whole
- Tapioca flour- 1 tablespoon

89

- pepper and salt to taste
- Twine
- Ice cubes- 4 cups
- Natural sugar replacement- 1 teaspoon
- Onions, chopped- 3
- Kosher salt- ½ cup
- xanthan gum- ½ teaspoon
- Celery cut into pieces- 4 stalks
- Sage- 1 bunch
- coarsely cracked black pepper divided- 1 ½ tablespoons
- Carrots cut into pieces, 4 carrots
- Water, divided- 2 gallons
- Fresh thyme leaves, chopped- 1 tablespoon
- Liquid fat in the form of ghee, bacon fat, or olive oil- ¼ cup
- Garlic cloves, crushed- 8
- Bay leaves- 3

INSTRUCTIONS:
1. The day before Thanksgiving, or whenever you are going to serve this turkey,you are going to get your turkey ready. Remove the bones and keep them aside.
2. Preheat your oven to 350 degrees Fahrenheit
3. Grease your roasting pan using whatever fat source you have chosen. Further, cover your turkey bones and the neck with 2 tablespoons of the fat. Put your bones on your roasting pan and put it into the preheated oven. This step is so that the turkey stock will have a more roasted taste.
4. Leave to roast for 30 minutes.

5. After 30 minutes has passed, flip them over and roast the other side for thirty more minutes. Check on them. They should have a more darkened color. If they seem to be pale, turn them over once again and cook them for 20 more minutes. Keep going in this way, until they golden brown. (you don't want to get them too dark, in order to avoid having a bitter taste).
6. Once the bones are done, take them out of the oven and put them into another big sized pot with a capacity of at least 2 gallons. Pour your water into the pot, enough to submerge the entirety. This will vary due to the size of your turkey, but you can expect somewhere around 5.5 liters of liquid.
7. Put this onto a large burner and turn the burner onto medium heat.
8. Deglaze the pan you used to roast the bones. Put the roasting pan on one or two hot burners, depending on its size, and add 1 cup of water. If you prefer, use white wine. Deglaze the pan using wine or water. Using a kitchen tool, remove any residue off of the bottom. Swirl to combine it into the liquid. A murky brown liquid will result.
9. Pour this liquid into pot containing the turkey broth.
10. Once turkey broth starts to simmer, lower the heat.
11. Simmer for 3 hours.
12. While simmering, come back to it on a recurring basis at 30 minute intervals. Use a large spoon to remove the top layer of the liquid in order to remove the fat, or that begins to accumulate at the top.
13. After 3 hours, put a big-sized cooking vessel on your burner on a high temperature level.
14. Put in some more of your fat of choice (around 1 tablespoon).

15. Next, put in your carrots. Mix them into the fat.
16. Cook the vegetables for long enough that they begin to get a browned in color.
17. Add 2 onions, diced. Add some salt and stir. Let heat up until they begin to caramelize.
18. Once they begin to caramelize, add them, along with the carrots to the turkey broth pot. At the same time, put in your bay leaf, your celery, and 1/2 of a tablespoon of pepper.
19. Take off the leaves of your sage stick and save the leaves to return to them again. Add the sage branches.
20. Leave it all cooking for one and a half hours.
21. Keep checking and skimming the top just like you did before.
22. Now we will make the brine. Take a big pot and boil 3 cups of water in it.
23. Sprinkle in 1/2 cup of salt. Stir and let it dissolve.
24. Take this off of the burner and put in the thyme, 2 bay leaves, the rest of the onion, garlic, and 1 tbsp of black pepper.
25. Leave this to sit for 15 minutes.
26. Get your ice and add enough water to make 5 cups of ice water.
27. Add your ice water into this. After the brine reduces in temperature quite a bit, put it in the refrigerator.
28. Return to your stock.
29. Strain the water off of the bones and other solids, so that the stock is then fully liquid. It will be about 1 gallon now. Throw out the bones and solids.
30. Place your stock in the fridge, uncovered overnight
31. Put your turkey leg meat and the breasts into your brine. Mix everything so that the meat is fully covered

by liquid. Leave this overnight as well, for at least 8 hours.

32. Place this into the refrigerator. Leave the turkey in the brine the turkey for somewhere around two to ten hours. No more than 12 hours.

33. The next day, you are going to reduce the turkey stock. Put it on the stovetop and bring it to a simmer. The goal is to reduce it by half. Once it gets to about half of the volume, remove 4 cups of it and leave this aside for other uses. Keep the other 4 cups on the stove and reduce this amount by half, once again. The last 2 cups will be what makes the gravy.

34. Remove also the turkey in the brine. Thoroughly rinse the turkey in cold water. Using paper towels, remove the excess water from it and set it to the side. You can get rid of the brine.

35. When you are ready to roast the turkey, preheat your oven to 450 degrees Fahrenheit.

36. Oil up your pan and put it off to the side.

37. Take a big baking sheet and, put one piece of bacon onto it. Then put another slice beside this one so that they are very slightly overlapping. Keep doing this, layering them over each other until you have a full sheet of raw bacon. This will take about 10 to 14 pieces of bacon.

38. Put your turkey legs on top of your bacon. Put the turkey legs beside each other. Put one half of your leaves that you took off of the sage branch on top of the legs. Lift up your bacon on one side and then roll it around the legs tightly. Using a spatula, gently move this roll to your roasting pan, which is ready off to the side.

39. Put one of the breasts, with the skin facing down, on the baking sheet and put on your remaining sage leaves. Then put the other turkey breast, skin side up, on top of the first breast, with the sage between them. Then use your twine to tie the roast. move it to the roasting pan with the legs already in it.

40. Put your pan into your preheated oven.

41. When about 14-16 mins have passed, lower the temperature to about 350 degrees Fahrenheit.

42. After 45 minutes have passed, check the temperature of the turkey with a thermometer. Put the thermometer in the deepest part of the breasts. It will probably need a little bit more time.

43. Measure the temperature every 10 minutes from this point on. Begin to pour the fat or the juices that have now collected in the bottom of the pan over top of the roasts.

44. The roast needs to cook for around 1 or 2 hours, depending on the size. When its internal temperature at the thickest part is 160 degrees Fahrenheit, take it out of the oven.

45. Put the roasts on a big platter and cover with foil, in a warm spot.

46. Rest them for around 20 minutes before you cut them.

47. Deglaze the pan you used for roasting with some water.

48. Put this pan over a burner, and as it heats up a little, remove the burnt pieces off of the bottom. Put this murky substance into your stock that you had set aside.

49. Take a new vessel and add your tapioca starch, your xanthan gum, your sweetener. Add a little bit of pepper and salt. Combine.
50. Place this reduced turkey stock on the stove on low heat. Add in the dry ingredients and whisk them. After whisking for some time, you will be able to tell how thick your gravy is.
51. If you want it to be thicker, make more of this dry mix. You can keep adjusting the thickness of your gravy until it's how you want it to be (be careful that you don't add too much, as you don't want to add carbohydrates to the nutritional facts.)
52. Taste the gravy, and adjust your level of seasoning until you are happy with it.
53. Slice your turkey. Add the gravy, and enjoy this delicious ketogenic festive meal.

Chapter 5: Weight Watchers Slow Cooker and Instant Pot Recipes

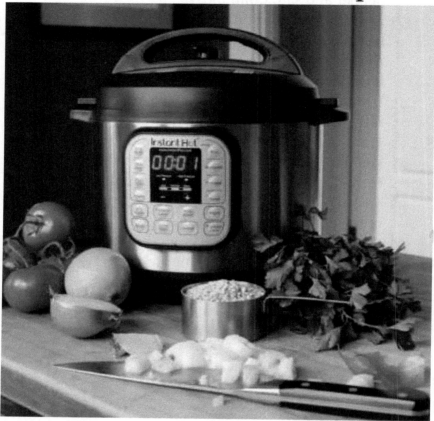

In this chapter, we are going to look at several recipes that can be prepared using an Instant Pot or using a Slow Cooker. We are going to first look at the science behind a slow cooker and an Instant Pot and how you can use either or both of these to make delicious, easy and simple dinners. For modern busy individuals, these two kitchen tools can change your life! They will not only provide you with great food every time, but they will help you stick to your Weight Watchers diet while cooking your food during your work day so that you come home to the smell of your dinner and all you had to do was put the ingredients into it and turn it on!

What Is an Instant Pot?

You have probably heard the term Instant Pot frequently as it is a new kitchen trend that has emerged internationally. If you are someone who is an avid cook, you likely are already familiar with what an instant pot does. However, unless you have actually used one, you probably don't realize the extent of its capabilities. It is a huge life-saver AND time-saver for the average busy household. Try to think of the instant pot as the opposite of a slow cooker. It is an electric pot that utilizes pressure to cook meals in a matter of minutes that would usually take hours on the stove. I will teach you about the different types of instant pots, what types of dishes you can cook with it, and some tips for you.

The Benefits of Using an Instant Pot

When purchasing an instant pot, it will come with standard features that are present in all models: warmer, yogurt maker, saute/browning, steamer, rice cooker, pressure cooker, and slow cooker. Advanced models of instant pots will also come with more features such as sterilizer, cake maker and egg maker. There are about twenty different models and sizes for Instant pots that range from 3 – 8 quartz. Some of these models even have wi-fi capabilities that will allow you to control and monitor the contents using your tablet or your phone.

If you are someone that works with many frozen ingredients and you don't have a lot of time on your hands, then the instant pot can help you with this. You can literally thaw foods straight from the freezer by following the right procedures. It is as simple as putting your frozen foods right into the pot, and it sautés them for a couple of minutes which will bring the temperature up. If you are trying to defrost cooked foods, you can also do this by steaming it in the instant pot without drying it out like the microwave would.

Some people often ask whether or not the instant pot will cause loss of ingredients in food. This is absolutely not true. This type of cooking actually allows the heat to be evenly distributed to all the foods so you wouldn't need to boil vegetables in water to thoroughly heat them, which is what usually causes the loss of nutrients. All you need is enough wonder to create steam and your food will be cooked like that.

Instant Pot Tips and Tricks

Although the instant pot sounds like magic right now, I do want to give you some tips when it comes to using them as mistakes CAN happen with it. First, food can be burnt using the instant pot. It is a bottom burner, so it means that if your pot doesn't have enough moisture, the bottom WILL burn. The other thing is that smells can become an issue as the pot uses a silicone ring to seal the lid. This is a great feature but if used overtime repeatedly, it can absorb orders and flavors of food. To avoid this, you just have to scrip the ring with baking soda and run it through the dishwasher. Not a hard fix but it will require attention. Lastly, the timer on the instant pot can be difficult to understand at first. There is a warm-up period that you have to account for before the actual timer kicks in. If you take all these tips into consideration, you should have an easy and fulfilling journey with your instant pot!

Top Instant Pot Mistakes to Avoid

Avoid these top mistakes to find Instant Pot Success!

1. Overfilling the Instant Pot
2. Forgetting to put the sealing ring back in the lid after cleaning
3. Using the rice button for any and all kinds of rice
4. Forgetting to turn the venting knob into the sealed position
5. Pressing the timer Button in an effort to Set the Cooking Time
6. Having too much liquid in the pot
7. A cooking liquid that is too thick
8. Placing the Instant Pot on the stovetop and accidentally turning on the stovetop!
9. Using the quick release button for foaming Foods or when it has been overfilled (see #1)
10. Not enough cooking liquid in the pot
11. Using hot liquid in a recipe that calls for cold liquid
12. Forgetting to put the inside pot back into the Instant Pot before you begin using it

Instant Pot Recipes and Cooking Times

In this section, you will find a variety of Instant Pot recipes for every occasion.

Instant Pot Tortilla Soup

Smart Points Value: 0 Smart Points Per Serving

INGREDIENTS:

- Boneless, Skinless Chicken Breasts- 2
- Canned or Frozen Corn- 8 ounces
- Black Beans, canned- 16 ounces
- Diced Tomatoes with Jalapenos, canned -16 ounces
- *You can also include your own fresh jalapeno peppers or other chilis to add spice if you wish.
- Crushed Tomatoes, Canned- 16 ounces
- Onion, diced- 1 large
- Garlic Powder- 1 tbsp
- Chicken Broth- 4 cups
- Chili Powder- 2 tsp
- Tortilla Strips- As many as you wish
- Cumin- 2 tsp
- Shredded Cheese, Sour Cream, Cilantro or any other toppings you want to put on to serve it

INSTRUCTIONS:
1   In your Instant Pot, put your beans, the corn, and your Onions and the diced tomatoes (with chilis or add the jalapenos separately at the same time)
2   Then, put in the chicken breasts

100

3 Sprinkle in the garlic powder, chili powder, and cumin

4 Next, pour in your crushed tomatoes and your chicken broth

5 Turn it on to manual high pressure

6 Cook for 30 minutes at this setting

7 Press Quick Release

8 Take the chicken out of the Instant Pot and shred it into small strips or pieces

9 Put your shredded chicken into the Instant Pot and mix everything together

10 Serve by putting your tortilla chips on top

11 This can be served with any toppings you wish, such as shredded cheese, sour cream, cilantro for topping, or any other toppings that you would normally put on your tacos!

Instant Pot Meatloaf

Smart Points Value: 11 Smart Points Per Serving

NUTRITIONAL INFORMATION:

Fat: 10 grams
Carbohydrates: 42 grams
Sugar: 10 grams
Fiber: 3 grams
Sodium: 566 grams
Protein: 31 grams
Calories: 380 calories
Serving size: 1 cup beans, 1/2 cup mashed potatoes, 1 slice meatloaf.
Serves: Makes 8 servings

MEATLOAF INGREDIENTS:
- Lean Ground Beef- 2 pounds
- Bread Crumbs- 1 Cup
- Eggs- 2
- Onion, Diced- ¼ of a cup
- Garlic Powder- 2 Teaspoons
- Parsley- 1 Teaspoon
- Barbeque Sauce- ½ of a cup
- Salt to taste
- Pepper to taste

SAUCE INGREDIENTS:
- Ketchup- ½ of a cup

- Brown Sugar- 2 tablespoons

POTATO INGREDIENTS:

- Medium-Sized Russet Potatoes, Cubed- 7
- Reduced Sodium Chicken Stock- 1 Cup
- Nonfat Milk- 1 Cup
- Garlic Powder- 2 teaspoons
- Pepper, to taste
- Salt, to taste

INSTRUCTIONS:
MEATLOAF:

1. In a bowl, combine your bread crumbs, the eggs, the garlic powder, ground beef, the onions, the barbeque sauce, the parsley and finally, the salt and pepper.
2. Put this meatloaf on a sheet of tinfoil.
3. Using your hands, begin to make the meat into the shape of a loaf. To do this, lift the sides of the tinfoil up around the meatloaf to shape it. This will also make it easier to move the loaf once it is cooked.
4. Wrap the tinfoil around the meatloaf

SAUCE:

1. To make your sauce, take a small bowl and add brown sugar and the ketchup
2. Mix this together until it is a homogenous mixture
3. Set this mix off to the side

POTATOES:

1. Remove the peel from the potatoes

2. Cut the peeled potatoes into small cubes.
3. Put these potatoes into your Instant Pot
4. Pour your chicken stock into the pot over the potatoes. Ensure that you have enough liquid in the pot so that nothing burns.
5. Take the wire rack attachment for the Instant Pot and put this over top of the potatoes.
6. Take the meatloaf that you have shaped and wrapped in foil and put this on the wire rack.
7. Put the lid on the Instant Pot.
8. Set the clock timer at 25 minutes and set the vent setting to "sealing."
9. Press the pressure cook button
10. After the time is up, let the pressure naturally release over the course of a 10-minute period
11. Open the Instant Pot and remove your meatloaf as well as the wire rack. You can use tongs to do this as it will be hot.
12. Take the sauce that you made and set aside and use a brush to glaze your meatloaf.
13. Let the meatloaf sit on the counter for 10 minutes.
14. Slice the meatloaf into slices and then plate it.
15. Leaving the potatoes in the Instant Pot, pour in your milk, as well as the salt, garlic powder, and pepper.
16. Once you have added these final ingredients, mash the warm potatoes using a potato masher.

Split Pea Soup With Ham

Smart Point Value: 1 Smart Point Per Serving
Calories- 182
Sugar- 4 grams
Fiber- 15 grams
Protein- 17 grams
Fat- 1.5 grams
Sodium- 459 mg
Carbohydrates- 39grams
Serving- 1 cup of soup

INGREDIENTS:
- Green Split Peas, Dry- 1 pound
- Olive Oil- 1 teaspoon
- Carrots, peeled - 2
- Onion, diced- 1
- Celery, diced- ¼ Cup
- Garlic, minced- 2 cloves
- Ham Bone Leftovers
- Water- 6 Cups
- Chicken Bouillon- 1 cube or 1 tablespoon
- Bay Leaf- 1 whole
- Ham, leftover, diced- 4 ounces
- Chives- to garnish with

INSTRUCTIONS:
1. Take your peas and run them under some cold water
2. In your Instant Pot, add the olive oil, carrots (diced), celery (diced), onions, and garlic (minced).
3. Set this to pressure sauté for somewhere between 3 to 5 minutes.

4. Add in the ham bone, the water, the peas, the bay leaf, and the chicken bouillon.
5. Replace the lid and cook all of this on the high pressure setting for about 15 minutes.
6. Let the pressure release itself naturally.
7. Open the lid and take out the bone and the bay leaf
8. Stir the soup that is left in the pot, and it should thicken naturally
9. If you wish, you can sauté your ham cubes on a stovetop skillet before adding them onto the soup as a garnish. Garnish your soup with chives also.
10. If you wish to try making this without an Instant Pot or pressure cooker, include 2 more cups of water and cook this on a low heat setting for 2 hours.

Vegan Mushroom Soup

Smart Points Value: 3 Points Per Serving

NUTRITIONAL INFORMATION:
Carbohydrates: 12.7g
Sodium: 738.2mg
Saturated Fat: 2.4g
Fat: 5.3g
Fiber: 3.6g
Protein: 4.8g
Sugar: 6.1g
Calories: 108.3kcal
Serving Size- 1.5 Cups of soup

INGREDIENTS:
- Olive Oil-2 teaspoons
- Onion, diced - 1
- Celery, diced- 1 Stalk
- Carrot, peeled & diced- 1
- Garlic, minced- 4 cloves
- Cremini Mushrooms, sliced- 4 ounces
- Shiitake Mushrooms, de-stemmed and sliced- 8 ounces
- Thyme, dried- 1 teaspoon
- Pepper- ½ of a teaspoon
- Vegetable Broth- 3 Cups
- Salt, Kosher- ½ of a teaspoon
- Coconut Milk- 2/3 of a cup

INSTRUCTIONS:
1. On your Instant Pot, turn the setting to Sauté mode.

2. Add in the olive oil, and once it is heated a little, then add the carrots, celery and the onion.
3. Sauté these vegetables in the pot.
4. Stir every now and then and cook it for 3 or 4 minutes or just until the vegetable begins to become softer.
5. Add both types of mushrooms as well as garlic, thyme and pepper.
6. Let this all cook together, infusing each element with the flavors of the others, and this stage will be done when the mushrooms begin to sweat out. This will take about 2 or 3 minutes.
7. Next, add in the vegetable broth as well as the salt.
8. Place the lid on the Instant Pot and close the steam vent. Then, set the pot to the manual high pressure setting.
9. Set the clock timer to 10 minutes. The Instant Pot will take about 10 minutes to reach its full high pressure setting.
10. When the 10-minute timer is up, use the quick release valve to let out the pressure, but be sure you are careful with this step to avoid an injury- it will be hot!
11. Remove half of the soup and put it into a blender To this, add half of the coconut milk.
12. Be sure to put a hand on the top of the blender lid and begin to blend this until it is just about smooth, ensuring that you leave some texture there still. NOTE: every now and then, stop the blender while blending and open the lid to release some steam as you are blending a hot substance.
13. Move this blended soup to a large bowl or a pot.
14. Take the second half of the soup out of the Instant Pot and put it into the blender, repeating the same process over again with the second half of the soup.

15. If you need to reheat the soup again at some point, you can do so by returning it to the Instant Pot and slowly heating it back up by setting the pot to Sauté mode once again.
16. Serve and enjoy!

Vegetarian Chili

Smart Points Value: 0 Smart Points Per Serving

NUTRITIONAL INFORMATION:
Calories- 34
Sodium- 577 mg
Carbohydrates- 6 grams
Fiber- 2 grams
Sugar- 3 grams
Protein- 1.5 grams

Serves: Makes 8 Servings

INSTRUCTIONS:
- Black beans- 1 can
- Tomatoes, Diced and canned- 20 ounces
- Onion, diced- 1
- Orange bell pepper, diced- one half
- Yellow bell pepper, diced- one half
- Green bell pepper, diced- one half
- Water- 5 C
- Vegetable bouillon- 2 cubes
- Black pepper- ½ of a tsp
- Cayenne powder- ½ of a tsp
- Chili powder- 2 tbsp
- Kidney beans- 1 can
- Garlic powder- 2 tsp
- Onion powder- 2 tsp
- Pinto beans- 1 can
- Dried oregano- 1 tsp
- Salt- 1 tsp

INSTRUCTIONS:
1. Put the Instant Pot onto the Sauté setting, and put in the oil, the bell peppers, and the diced onion.
2. Let them sauté for about 5 minutes, or just until they begin to soften
3. Put in the pinto beans, the black beans, the diced tomatoes, and the kidney beans.
4. Sprinkle in all of the seasonings, including the cayenne powder, the chili powder, the garlic powder, the onion powder, the salt and the dried oregano, as well as the 5 cups of water. Then, stir everything well in order to combine it.
5. Put the lid on your Instant Pot and put it on to the seal setting.
6. Cook this on the Manual High Pressure setting for about fifteen minutes.
7. Let the steam escape over the course of 10 minutes.
8. Then serve this with any toppings you like on your chili such as sour cream, green onions, lime pieces or lime juice, cilantro, avocado, and cheese.

**Buffalo Chicken Lettuce Wraps**

Smart Points Value: 0 Smart Points Per Serving

NUTRITIONAL INFORMATION:
Serves- Makes 3 cups of chicken
Serving Size- 1/2 cup

Fat: 0 grams
Carbohydrates: 5.5 grams
Protein: 24 grams
Sodium: 879 milligrams
Fiber: 12 grams
Sugar: 2 grams
Calories: 148 kcal

INGREDIENTS:
- Boneless, Skinless Chicken Breasts- 3
- Celery stalk, diced- 1
- Onion, diced- One Half
- Garlic, minced- 1 clove
- Chicken Broth, Fat-Free, Low-Sodium- 16 ounces
- Cayenne pepper sauce or other hot sauce- 16 ounces

Wrap Ingredients:
- Lettuce leaves- 6 Large sized leaves
- Carrots, shredded- 1 and ½ Cups
- Celery Stalk, Sliced into small matchstick shapes - 2 large stalks

INSTRUCTIONS:

This recipe can be done using either a slow cooker or an instant pot, whichever you wish to use will work well, but the instructions will be slightly different. Below, you can see both of the recipes for these two options.

The Slow Cooker Method

1. In your slow cooker, put in the chicken breasts, the celery stalk, the onions, the minced garlic, and the chicken broth.
2. Make sure that your chicken broth is enough to cover the chicken breasts. If not, you can add some water to the broth in order to cover the chicken breasts.
3. Put the lid on and cook this at a high setting for a duration of 4 hours of cooking time.
4. Remove the chicken from the pot.
5. Take out also 1/2 of a cup of broth from the slow cooker and set it aside. You can discard the rest of the broth.
6. Then, shred the chicken using a knife or fork and then put it back into the slow cooker, as well as your reserved one-half cup of broth. Add the hot sauce to the pot as well and then turn the slow cooker setting to "high" and cook this for 30 more minutes.
7. While this is cooking, get your lettuce wraps ready. To do this, put ¼ of a cup of carrots, any dressing you wish, and the celery matchsticks into the lettuce wrap.
8. When the chicken is finished, add this to your lettuce wraps, and then they are ready!
9. Wrap up and start eating!

The Instant Pot Method:

1. In your Instant Pot, put in the chicken breasts, the celery stalk, the onions, the minced garlic, and the chicken broth. Make sure that your chicken broth is enough to cover the chicken breasts. If not, you can add some water to the broth in order to cover the chicken breasts.

2. Cover your Instant Pot with the lid and turn it on to its high pressure setting for 15 minutes. Then, allow it to naturally release.

3. Take the chicken out of the pot.

4. Take out also 1/2 of a cup of broth from the Instant Pot and set it aside. You can discard the rest of the broth.

5. Then, shred the chicken using a knife or with two forks and then return it to the Instant Pot, along with the one-half cup of broth that you set aside previously.

6. Add the hot sauce to the pot as well and then turn the Instant Pot to the sauté setting. Sauté for 2 to 3 minutes.

7. While this is cooking, get your lettuce wraps ready. To do this, put ¼ of a cup of carrots, any dressing you wish, and the celery matchsticks into the lettuce wrap.

8. When the chicken is finished, add this to your lettuce wraps, and then they are ready!

9. Wrap up and start eating!

Chicken and Dumplings

Smart Points Value: 5 Smart Points Per Serving

NUTRITIONAL INFORMATION:
Serving Size: 1 -2/3 cups soup along with 4 dumplings
Calories-276
Sugar 6g
Carbohydrates 38g
Protein 21g
Saturated Fat 1 gram
Sodium 979mg
Cholesterol 38mg
Calories from Fat 45
Fat 5g
Fiber 2g

INGREDIENTS:
- Frozen Corn- 1 Cup
- Carrots, diced- 1 Cup
- Celery, diced- 3 or 4 stalks
- Chicken Broth, Fat- Free- 5 Cups
- Boneless, Skinless Chicken Breasts- 1 pound
- Bisquick Baking Mix- 2 cups
- Nonfat Milk- 1 cup
- Frozen Peas (optional) - 1 cup
- Parsley, Fresh (optional)
- Pepper and Salt to taste

INSTRUCTIONS:

1. In your Instant Pot, add the carrots, the celery and the corn. Then, add your chicken broth into the pot as well.
2. Next, add your chicken breast to the Instant Pot.
3. Set the Instant Pot to the HIGH level and put the timer setting to 10 minutes (if your chicken is being cooked from frozen) or 8 minutes (if your chicken has already been thawed).
4. Take a small size bowl and add in the Bisquick and the milk, and then leave this off to the side.
5. Press the quick release button when the full allotted time has elapsed in order to let the pressure out.
6. Remove the lid from the Instant Pot, however, leave the pot onto the HIGH heat setting.
7. Take the chicken out of the pot and using a knife or two forks, begin to shred it into small pieces.
8. If you are going to be adding peas into this recipe, this is where you will add them in.
9. Put the chicken back into the Instant Pot, but be careful that you do not burn yourself or splash yourself with the hot broth when you do this.
10. Go back to your Bisquick mixture and spoon scoops of this into the broth one tablespoon at a time to make your biscuits.
11. Let your dumplings cook for about 8 or 10 minutes on high heat until the dumplings become dumplings! At about 4 or 5 minutes, flip the dumplings over so that they cook evenly.
12. Turn off the Instant Pot, and your chicken and dumplings are ready to serve!
13. Add Salt and pepper to taste as you wish.
14. Sprinkle some parsley on top if you wish.

Cilantro Lime Quinoa With Chipotle Chicken

Smart Points Value: 8 Smart Points Per Serving

CHICKEN INGREDIENTS:
- Salt, Kosher- 1/2 teaspoon
- Cumin, Ground- 1/2 teaspoon
- Black pepper- for taste
- Chipotle Paste- 1 tablespoon
- Mild Salsa- 1 cup
- Boneless, Skinless Chicken Thighs- 1 pound
- Corn on the cob- 2 ears

QUINOA INGREDIENTS:
- Quinoa, uncooked, rinsed and drained- 3/4 cup
- Water- 1 cup as well as an additional 2 tablespoons
- Salt, Kosher- 1/4 teaspoon
- The juice of 1 lime
- Olive oil- 1/2 tablespoon
- Chopped Cilantro- 2 tablespoons

BOWL INGREDIENTS:
- Cherry Tomatoes, Halved- 1 cup
- Avocado, sliced- 1 small
- Lime- 4 wedges
- Chopped Cilantro- 2 tablespoons

INSTRUCTIONS:

1. Take a bowl and in it, put the cumin, the black pepper, the salt, the chipotle, and the salsa.
2. Put the chicken in your Instant Pot and put the salsa over top of the chicken.
3. Cook this on the high pressure setting for about 20 minutes. When this time has elapsed, you can use either the Quick release or the natural release.
4. Add the corn and then cook this on high pressure for another 2 minutes.
5. While this is cooking, put your quinoa, water, and the salt into a small pot and cook this on high heat on your stovetop. Let this come to a boil.
6. When the quinoa is boiling, reduce your temperature and then put a cover on your pot.
7. Cook the quinoa for around 17 to 23 minutes, or just until the liquid has all been absorbed.
8. When it is finished, fluff it up using a fork and take it off of the heat.
9. Add in the olive oil, the lime juice as well as 1/4 cup of cilantro. Stir to combine it.
10. When the chicken has finished cooking, take out the corn, and put it off to the side.
11. Also, take out the chicken and put it in a bowl. Then, shred it using two forks.
12. Add 1/2 cup of the sauce to this shredded chicken in the bowl.
13. Use a knife to cut the corn off of the husk.
14. Put 2/3 cup of quinoa in a bowl, along with 1/2 cup of shredded chicken. Put some more sauce on top if you wish, as well as 1/3 cup corn, 1/4 cup tomatoes, and 1-ounce avocado. This will make up one serving according to the recipe.

15. Put the remaining cilantro on top of the serving and serve this all with the lime wedges.

Turkey Stroganoff

Smart Points Value: 7 Smart Points Per Serving

INGREDIENTS:
- Olive oil, divided- 1 teaspoon
- Onion, diced- 1/2 cup
- Ground Turkey- 1 pound
- Whole Wheat Seasoned Bread Crumbs- 1/3 cup
- Egg, beaten- 1 Large Size
- Parsley, chopped- 1/4 cup
- Fat-Free Milk- 3 tablespoons
- Salt, Kosher- 3/4 tsp
- Black Pepper, for taste
- Water- 3/4 cups
- Light Sour Cream- 1/2 cup
- All-Purpose Flour- 2 tbsp
- Tomato paste- 2 teaspoons
- Beef Bouillon- 2 teaspoons
- Worcestershire sauce- 1/2 teaspoon
- Paprika - 1/2 teaspoon
- Cremini mushrooms, Sliced- 8 ounces
- Thyme, Fresh- 1 sprig

INSTRUCTIONS:
1. Turn on your Instant Pot to its sauté setting and spray it with some oil
2. Sauté your onions in the Instant Pot until they become softened and golden brown. Stir them while they cook for about 2 to 3 minutes.

3. Take the onions out of the pot and divide the portion in two.

4. Take a big bowl and add in one half of the sautéed onions along with 2 tbsp of the parsley, the bread crumbs, the ground turkey, the egg, milk, 3/4 tsp of salt and as much black pepper as you want.

5. Using your hands, combine all of this together and then begin to make the shapes of about 20 meatballs.

6. To the side, in a blender, blend together the tomato paste, sour cream, the water, flour, the beef bouillon, Worcestershire sauce, and paprika. Continue to blend it until it becomes smooth.

7. Set your pot on to the sauté setting again, then add your oil and half of the meatballs. Begin to brown them without touching them. Cook them for about 2 minutes; you will know when they are done if they no longer stick to the pot. When this occurs, turn them over and brown the other side for another 2 minutes.

8. Put the first half of the cooked meatballs onto a clean plate and cook the second half of them.

9. Then, put all of the meatballs as well as the remaining onion into the Instant Pot, and then add the sauce over top of the meatballs, as well as the thyme and the mushrooms.

This recipe can be finished in several ways, and they are each outlined below for you, depending on what you prefer to finish it off with.

Using The Instant Pot:

Cook this on the high pressure setting for 10 minutes. Allow the pressure to release on its own, naturally.

Using The Stove Top:

Add 2 tablespoons of water and bring it to a boil. Then, cook this covered by a lid on low heat for 20 to 25 minutes.

When it is done, remove the thyme, and then add in the chopped parsley. You can then serve this over top of any type of noodles.

Using The Slow Cooker:

Cook in the slow cooker on the low setting for 6 to 8 hours.

When it is done, remove the thyme, and then add in the chopped parsley. You can then serve this over top of any type of noodles.

Beef Barbacoa

Smart Points Value: 3 Smart Points Per Serving

INGREDIENTS:
- Garlic- 5 cloves
- Medium onion- 1/2 of one
- The juice of one lime
- Chipotles in adobo sauce, to taste- 2-4 tbsp
- Ground cumin- 1 tbsp
- Ground oregano- 1 tbsp
- Ground cloves- 1/2 tsp
- Water- 1 cup
- Beef eye with the fat removed - 3 lbs
- Salt, Kosher - 2 1/2 teaspoons
- black pepper to taste
- Oil, of your choice- 1 tsp
- Bay Leaves- 3

INSTRUCTIONS:
1. Put the lime juice, chipotles, the cumin, the garlic, the onion, the oregano, cloves, and water into a blender and blend this on the puree setting until it becomes a smooth mixture.
2. Remove all of the fat from the meat, and then slice it so that it is in slices of about 3-inches each.
3. Rub the meat slices with both salt and black pepper.
4. Turn on your Instant Pot to the sauté setting. When it heats up enough, add in the oil and the meat.
5. Begin to brown the meat, in as many batches as you need to. Brown it on every side, which takes around 5 mins for every set.

6. Take your sauce from the blender as well as the bay leaves and add this to the Instant Pot. Cover the pot and cook on the high pressure setting until all of the meat is tender, and it will easily shred. This will take about one hour. When finished, use the Natural release method to allow the pressure to escape.

7. You can shred the meat using 2 forks.

8. When it has finished cooking and has become tender, take your meat out of the pot and shred it.

9. Reserve the liquid that is in the Instant Pot for later, but you can get rid of your bay leaf.

10. Put the beef back into your Instant Pot, and then add as much salt as you wish to taste, as well as one half teaspoon of cumin, 1 1/2 cups of the juice that you kept from before.

11. Then, mix it all together, and it is ready to be served! You can eat this over rice with fresh herbs or in a wrap or burrito! Get creative with this!

Pulled Pork

Smart Points Value: 1 Smart Point Per Serving

INGREDIENTS:
Roasted Red Peppers- 1 Small can
Bay leaf- 2
1 tsp olive oil
1 teaspoon kosher salt
black pepper, to taste
Parsley, Fresh- 1 Tablespoon
Crushed Tomatoes- 1 Can
Garlic- 5 cloves

Thyme, Fresh- 2 sprigs
18 oz pork tenderloin

INSTANT POT METHOD:

1. Rub the pork tenderloin using pepper and salt.
2. Turn the Instant Pot onto the sauté setting to warm it up.
3. Add your garlic as well as your oil and sauté them long enough to become browned, which will take somewhere between 1 and 1 1/2 minutes.
4. Remove them from the pot with a slotted spoon.
5. Add the pork and brown it in the pot for only roughly two and a half minutes for each side.
6. Put in the rest of the ingredients as well as your browned garlic but be sure to reserve half of the parsley.
7. Cook on the high pressure setting for 45 minutes.
8. Use the Natural release method when finished.
9. Remove the bay leaf.
10. Pull apart the pork using a fork and put the rest of the parsley for garnish.
11. This can be eaten with pasta, in a burrito, on rice or any other way you like.

SLOW COOKER METHOD:

1. Rub the pork tenderloin using pepper and salt.
2. Take a frying pan and warm it up on medium to high.
3. Toss in the garlic and pour in your oil and cook it for about one or two minutes, until browned.
4. Take out the garlic from the pan.

5. Put the pork into the skillet and begin to cook it for about two or three mins per side.
6. Take it out and put the pork into the slow cooker. Add in the rest of the ingredients as well as the browned garlic. Reserve half of the parsley for later.
7. Cook this in the slow cooker for 8 hours on a low setting.
8. Remove the bay leaves.
9. Shred the pork with 2 forks and top it with remaining parsley. Serve over your favorite pasta, in a burrito, on rice or any other way you like.

Spaghetti and Meat Sauce

Smart Points Value: 10 Smart Points Per Serving

NUTRITIONAL INFORMATION:
Serving: 1 and ½cups
Calories: 392kcal
Carbohydrates: 45 grams
Protein: 24 grams
Fat: 15 grams
Cholesterol: 63.5 mg
Sodium: 740 mg
Fiber: 6 grams
Sugar: 6.5 grams

INGREDIENTS:
- Ground Turkey- 1 pound
- Salt, Kosher - 3/4 teaspoon
- Onion, diced - 1/4 cup
- Garlic, minced- 1 clove
- Your favorite tomato sauce jar- 1 25-ounce jar
- Water- 2 cups
- Whole wheat spaghetti- 8 ounces
- Grated parmesan cheese, optional for serving

INSTRUCTIONS:
1. Put your Instant Pot onto the sauté setting. When it is hot enough, add the turkey and the salt and cook it, being sure to break it up as it cooks. This will take about 3 minutes to cook.

2. Add in the onions, and garlic and cook until they become softened, which will take about 3 to 4 minutes.
3. Add the tomato sauce jar, the water, and the spaghetti (break the spaghetti in half before adding it in). Make sure that the liquid covers everything in the pot without you having to stir it.
4. Cover it with the lid and cook it on high pressure for 9 minutes.
5. Quick release this so that the pasta doesn't continue to cook and serve it, topped with grated parmesan cheese if desired!

Mashed Potatoes

Smart Points Value: 5 Smart Points Per Serving

NUTRITIONAL INFORMATION:
Serving: 3/4 cup

Fat: 4g
Protein: 5g
Sodium: 324mg
Cholesterol: 11.5mg
Calories: 142kcal
Saturated Fat: 2.5g
Sugar: 3.5g
Fiber: 3g
Carbohydrates: 27g

INGREDIENTS:
- Russet potatoes, quartered and peeled- 2 pounds
- Water- 3 cups
- Salt, Kosher- 1/2 teaspoon
- Low-fat 1% buttermilk- 1/3 cup
- Light sour cream- 1/4 cup
- Whipped butter- 2 tablespoons
- Salt, Kosher- 1 teaspoon
- Black pepper, to taste
- Chopped chives for garnish
- Chopped parsley for garnish

INSTRUCTIONS:

1. Add your potatoes to your Instant Pot and pour enough water to just cover them all. Then, season them with salt.
2. Cover the pot with the lid and then cook the potatoes on the high pressure setting for 10 minutes.
3. Use the quick release function to check if the potatoes are soft. You will know that they are done when a sharp knife can slide through them with ease.
4. Drain the water off of the potatoes, but reserve 1/2 cup of the cooking water.
5. Add in the butter, the buttermilk, and the sour cream, as well as the salt and the black pepper to the hot potatoes. Then, mash all of this with a potato masher.
6. Taste them and adjust the salt level to taste.
7. Keep them in the pot on the warm setting until you are ready to serve them.
8. They are best when served right away, but if you need to leave them to eat them later, you can use the cooking water that you put aside to rehydrate them if they dry out.
9. Serve them with the chopped chives and or parsley to garnish them on top.

Garlic and Parmesan Artichokes

Smart Points Value: 3 Smart Points Per Serving

NUTRITIONAL INFORMATION:
Calories: 127kcal

Carbohydrates: 15 Grams
Protein: 7 grams
Fat: 5 grams
Saturated Fat: 2 grams
Sodium: 215 mg
Fiber: 7 grams
Sugar: 0.5 grams
Vitamin C: 16 mg
Calcium: 129 mg
Iron: 2 mg

- INGREDIENTS:
  Artichokes- 4
  Garlic, Minced- 2 tsp
  Olive oil- 4 tsp
  Parmesan cheese, grated or shredded - 1/4 cup
  Chicken broth or Vegetable broth- ½ Cup (you could also use water if you prefer or if it is all you have on hand)

INSTRUCTIONS:

1. Wash your artichokes and trim them so that you are removing the top of the artichoke, as well as the outer leaves and the stem.

2. Spread each artichoke open using your hands and into the top of each one add 1/2 teaspoon of the minced garlic.
3. Drizzle 1 tsp of olive oil over top of them as well.
4. Sprinkle each artichoke with 1 tbsp of grated or shredded parmesan cheese.
5. Using the basket insert for you Instant Pot, put your artichokes into the Instant Pot on the basket.
6. Pour in 1/2 cup of the water, or the chicken or vegetable broth- whichever you chose.
7. Seal the Instant Pot with the lid and make sure that the valve is set to the seal setting.
8. Select the steam option on the pot and cook the artichokes for 10 minutes.
9. If you have smaller artichokes, you will maybe need to reduce the cooking time by a couple of minutes.
10. Once the cooking time has completed, use the quick release method to let the steam out of the pot by moving the valve to the venting setting.
11. Remember to use an oven mitt in order to protect your hands from the very hot steam.
12. Plate them and serve!

Slow Cooker Recipes

As you have seen, some of the recipes included in the previous section could be completed either using an Instant Pot or a Slow Cooker. In this section, we will look at some more slow cooker-specific recipes that you can try!

Slow Cooker Chicken Cacciatore

Smart Points Value: 0 Smart Points Per Serving

NUTRITIONAL INFORMATION:

Prep Time- 30 minutes
Cook Time- 4 hours
Total Time- 4 hours and 30 minutes
Servings- 8 servings
Calories- 311kcal
Serving: 1 serving contains the following,

Sugar: 5 g
Calcium: 48 mg
Fiber: 2g
Iron: 3 mg
Fat: 21 g
Sodium: 445 mg
Calories: 311kcal
Protein: 22 grams
Carbohydrates: 11 grams

INGREDIENTS:
- Bone-In Skinless Chicken Thighs, Fat-Trimmed - 8
- Salt, Kosher - 3/4 teaspoon

- Oregano- 1 stick
- Black pepper to taste
- Oil or spray for nonstick feature
- Onion, finely chopped- 1/2 of one large onion
- Crushed tomatoes- One 28-ounce can
- Red bell pepper, chopped- 1/2
- Green bell pepper, chopped- 1/2
- Shiitake mushrooms- 4 ounces
- Thyme- 1 stick
- Garlic cloves, finely chopped- 5
- Bay leaf- 1
- Parsley, chopped- 1 tablespoon (optional)
- Parmesan cheese, freshly grated (optional as a garnish)

INSTRUCTIONS:
1. Rub your chicken using some salt and pepper.
2. Warm a big enough pan on med-high.
3. Season the pan using oil and put in your chicken.
4. Cook this until it begins to change color- which will take about three minutes each side.
5. Transfer the chicken to your slow cooker. (If you decided to use chicken breast instead, you can skip this step and put the chicken directly into the slow cooker with salt and pepper).
6. Put this in for 6 hours in the slow cooker on low heat or for 2 to 3 hours on high heat, if you are using chicken breasts.
7. Go back to your nonstick pan and bring the heat level down to medium. Coat the pan with more oil.

8. Put in the onion and garlic to the pan and sauté it, stirring it occasionally, until it becomes soft- this will take about 3 to 4 minutes.
9. Transfer the garlic and onion to the slow cooker and then also add the thyme, bell peppers, tomatoes, mushrooms, oregano, and bay leaf to the slow cooker. Stir to combine everything.
10. Cover the slow cooker and cook this on high heat for 4 hours or on low heat for 8 hours.
11. Get rid of your leaf and move your chicken over to a big enough plate.
12. Take the chicken meat off of the bones and get rid of the bones. Then, shred the chicken meat, and put it back into the sauce.
13. Stir in the parsley (if you have decided to use it).
14. If you want, serve this dish topped with Parmesan cheese.

NOTES:

- If you wish to be more strict with your Weight Watchers points, make this recipe instead with 1 and 1/2 to 2 pounds of boneless, skinless chicken breast instead of the thighs.
- If you need this recipe to be gluten-free, make sure that you use a can of tomatoes that is also Gluten Free, as this is often a hidden source of gluten.

Slow Cooker Chicken Vegetable Soup

Smart Points Value: 0 Smart Points Per Serving

Preparation Time: 20 Minutes
Cooking Time: 7 Hours
Total Time: 7 Hours and 20 Minutes

Calories: 150

INGREDIENTS:
- Black pepper- 1/8 teaspoon
- Dried thyme leaves- 1 teaspoon
- Boneless, skinless chicken breast- 1 and 1/2 pounds
- Onion, finely diced - 1/2 cup
- Carrots, chopped- 2
- Dry coleslaw mix (shredded cabbage and carrots)- 3 cups
- Chicken broth- 2 cans
- White kidney beans, drained - 1 can
- Stewed tomatoes, not drained- 1 can
- Salt- 1/2 teaspoon
- Frozen peas- 1 cup
- Bay leaf- 1

INSTRUCTIONS:
1. This recipe was made with a slow cooker size of 6-Quarts.
2. To begin, evenly rub the chicken breasts with 1/4 tsp of pepper and salt

3. Put all of the ingredients in the crockpot and stir them to combine them.
4. Cover with the lid and cook everything on the HIGH setting for 3 to 4 hours, or instead on LOW for about 6 to 8 hours, you will know that it is done when the vegetables are softened, and the chicken is white on the inside.
5. Take out your bay leaf.
6. Remove the chicken and put it on a plate.
7. Pull each chicken breast with a fork.
8. Put the chicken back into the slow cooker and stir the chicken into the soup.
9. Season the soup to taste as you wish, and it is ready to serve!

Conclusion

Before you begin your WW program, there are some things that you will want to do to prepare yourself. This new journey you are embarking on may be difficult mentally and physically, especially if you are new to following a specific diet plan. Your mindset will become very important as you begin, especially as you get deeper into the program. Getting yourself into the proper mindset before you begin will help you to stay focused when the going gets tough.

How to Keep Yourself Motivated & on Track

When it comes to finding motivation in those tough moments, it will come down to the reasons that made you want to begin this journey in the first place.

Everybody's objective will differ slightly and will likely be quite personal to them. Maybe you want to reduce your risk of cancer because it runs in your family. Maybe you have been obese for the majority of your life, and you are trying this as a means of weight loss and health improvement. Maybe you heard about it and challenged yourself to try it for a few months to see how it feels. Whatever your objective, writing it down will help to solidify it and make it real. Then, when you are wondering why on earth you decided to put yourself through this on the first day of your new diet plan, you can look at that objective that you wrote down, and it will re-inspire you to continue. When it comes to mindset, being aware of your motivation is extremely beneficial.

When it comes to something like dieting, the mental game is the biggest part of it. You already know that your body can survive a new diet and a new lifestyle. You know that you will be getting the nutrients you need from the food that you will eat. You know that your body will likely even feel better for having changed your diet. What all this means is that the part that makes this new lifestyle and diet plan very difficult is the mental part. During a big life change, the mindset will play a huge part in how you feel and how you remain motivated throughout your journey.

Success depends on whether or not a person has a growth mindset. A fixed mindset is when a person believes that their intelligence and skills are a fixed trait. They have what they have, and that's it. This makes the person highly concerned with what skills and intelligence they currently have, and they do not focus on what they can gain. Therefore, their activities are limited to the capacity that they think they have. However, those with growth mindsets understand that skills and intelligence is something that can be developed and learned throughout the course of their life. This can be done through education, training, or simply just even passion. They understand that their brain is a muscle that can be 'worked out' to grow stronger.

Knowing this, it is important that you employ a growth mindset. Every single skill you have, and anything that you wish to try or to improve upon can be ameliorated by putting in the effort to see it from a growth mindset. This is the mindset for success when it comes to life in general, but especially when it comes to changing something about your lifestyle- like beginning an intermittent fasting regimen.

Think about what mindset you have right now. If you already have a growth mindset, you simply need to continue practicing it while being proactive about avoiding obstacles and overcoming failures. If you think you are someone with a fixed mindset, change it right now. Believe me when I tell you that intelligence and skills can be improved upon with time and hard work. If you don't believe me, just try it. Pick a random skill; this could be knitting, programming, jogging, or anything that can be learned. Set goals for yourself and begin learning something new. If you are able to take something that you have zero skill in and become proficient in it, you have just proved to yourself that growth mindsets are real and fixed mindsets only hold you back from success.

What to Do If You Fall Off Track

When it comes to following a new lifestyle plan, it is important to ensure that you approach it in a way that will be beneficial for your health, and that it will not do any harm to your body, as the purpose of this new lifestyle is to reach a healthy state of body and mind. In this section, we will look at what you should do if you find yourself falling off track.

Firstly, you want to maintain flexibility with yourself and your body when dieting. For example, if you are not feeling well one day, and the diet is feeling more difficult than other days for some reason, don't be afraid to make a change that day that will help you to feel better both mentally and physically. This is especially true at the beginning when you first introduce this new diet into your life. If you have your mind set on a specific plan, where you will omit certain foods that you are used to eating, you may find it difficult at first. In order to help yourself to get over the difficult adjustment phase, you can remain flexible with your mind and body in order to keep yourself in a good mental state.

Maintaining this flexible mindset will allow you to remain healthy, and it will allow you to pay more attention to how you are feeling than to the plan that you have set out for yourself. As you get more comfortable with the diet and lifestyle, you can then begin to become a little more rigid and strict, as long as you do so in a gradual manner, in order to keep yourself feeling positive about the journey.

Mindset for Successful Dieting & Weight Loss

What you choose to focus on during your fast will determine if you are having a terrible time and counting down the hours until you can eat again, or if you barely notice them going by. By focusing on what you are depriving yourself of you will see everything as a punishment, you are putting yourself through. This will make it very difficult for you to make it through your fasting period as everything except water and coffee will seem like it has been placed before your eyes to punish you. By instead looking at the things that you are giving yourself- like tea, black coffee, and water and appreciating these things, it will help you to rediscover how refreshing and nourishing water is, a fact that we take for granted in places where our water is clean and drinkable. You will be able to taste the coffee beans without the cream and sugar that cover up their beauty. You will be able to appreciate the tea leaves that spend time growing in order to end up in this cup of yours. You will also appreciate your food that much more when you reach your eating window, and you can eat whatever you want. By viewing your day through the lens of appreciation instead of deprivation, you will have a much easier time with your fast.

141

By expecting that there will be some uncomfortable side-effects such as cravings, hunger, and irritability, you can greet them with the feeling of "Oh hello, I have been expecting you." Rather than "Oh no, I am feeling so terrible, what is going on?" If you are not surprised that you will feel a little bit uncomfortable while your body adapts to your new diet, you will be able to greet it- rather than fight it, which will make you much more comfortable with it all.

It is important to recognize when following this new diet plan, that this is a choice you are making for your health, your body, or whatever specific objective you have. You must recognize that this is a choice you are consciously making and that you have decided to go through this new lifestyle change in order to receive the benefits later. If you lose sight of the fact that this is a choice you are making, you may begin to feel like a victim or like the universe is punishing you. This victim mindset will only make things harder for you. By taking responsibility for your decision to follow this plan, you will not allow yourself to slip into this negative mindset and will instead feel confident and in control of your decision. This will help you to view things through the lens of appreciation rather than deprivation like I outlined above.

You can prepare as much as you like, but while you are dieting, you could be met with some unexpected feelings. Challenging your body and mind often brings up many feelings for us, as it puts us in a state of self-reflection and deep thought. This is normal. Think about if you decided to run a marathon. While running, as your legs desperately want to give up and your body is tired, your mind will likely go to some deep places that they do not go when you are going about your regular daily duties. Dieting is similar to the marathon in this way, as it can be very challenging for both the body and the mind.

When emotions come up during your diet and your change in lifestyle , it is important to know what to do with them. The first step is to acknowledge them. By acknowledging these emotions, you can tap into them and examine them in more depth. The next step is to write them down. This can be a very quick note of how you are feeling or what is the most challenging part for you. By writing it down, you are processing this emotion, and you are able to address it instead of pushing it away. When we push our emotions away, they do not really go away; they just go dormant for a short period of time only to come up later. By addressing them, you can examine what is going on inside of you.

As you begin your new diet, keep a small journal with you so that you can write down notes about how you are feeling. Even if you don't have the time to examine your feelings deeply, write them down so that you can come back to them later in order to look into them more deeply. This will help you to process them and keep a record of them so that you can better understand yourself, especially as you go through changes.

Lightning Source UK Ltd.
Milton Keynes UK
UKHW050808010221
378038UK00005B/60